If I Could, I Would

If I Could, I Would

AN INSPIRING STORY OF A
YOUNG GIRL WHO LIVED
LIFE TO THE FULLEST

• • •

H. Russel Lemcke

ISBN-13: 9781496113894
ISBN-10: 1496113896
Library of Congress Control Number: 2017901680
CreateSpace Independent Publishing Platform
North Charleston, South Carolina

Contents

Net revenue from the sale of this book will go to not for profit organizations helping the under privileged.

Preface

● ● ●

IF THIS WERE ONLY THE story of the death of a nineteen-year-old, it would not have been written. This is a story of courage in life and courage in facing death. And it is a story about the continuity of life.

This book is also the fulfillment of a promise. Stephanie came to understand after a lot of reaffirmation that she was unique. She also came to believe that she could help others by telling her story. Her death did not permit the story to be written by her. But my pen, perhaps guided by her spirit, is second-best. The title If I Could, I Would is from the U2 song "Bad" which was particularly meaningful to her.

Woven within the words is the revelation by a father that parents can be educated about life, death and courage by a child they previously may have thought it was their job to teach.

At time of publishing, thirty years have passed since Stephanie passed away. The book has been written and rewritten three times, each time with more memories and probably greater introspection. The first pass was rather short, instructional, and not substantive. I never felt angry about her condition but felt the need early on to tell people about her rather than let her words speak for themselves. Time has changed that perspective. However, the pain associated with her difficult life and untimely death has not fully subsided. I am often reminded of what our pastor said at her graveside. He explained the pain of loss in terms of an old 33⅓ RPM record, saying grief is like that record. It seems at the start that it will go on forever, but over time the end of the pain seems closer than the start. And after a time, one does not want the pain to completely go away, as that could imply full loss of the loved one. After all these years, that 33⅓ record keeps on playing.

Prologue

● ● ●

FOR ANYONE WHO HAS FLOWN in the Boeing 747, the sensation is the same. Takeoff seems all too slow—almost animated. Likewise for climb out—the scenes below seem to pass by in slow motion. And so it was on this sparkling clear evening of May 10, 1986 at John F. Kennedy Airport in New York as Aer Lingus flight 104 seemed to push the ground away and begin its methodical ascent. Gaining altitude, the shamrock-labeled jumbo jet made a slow, almost suspended turn over Long Island Sound, leveled its wings, and then deliberately gained power. As we continued our ascent, I permitted myself to recline my seat. I could feel strain subside from my neck muscles. I realized I had been filled with tension for a long time.

In the window and aisle seats immediately in front of me were my eighteen-year-old daughter, Stephanie, and her friend Marya. We were on our way to Dublin, Ireland, a trip arranged with great speed and created out of a deep desire to do something—anything—to help keep Stephanie's life whole. To Stephanie, it was so much. To me, so little compared with the life I desperately wanted to keep. And yet I knew even then that we were losing.

Sleep evaded me during the Atlantic crossing. Many thoughts of our upcoming private lunch with the now world-famous Irish rock group U2 occupied my mind. What if the arrangements resulted in a superficial, brief encounter? I had visions of us sitting at a booth for six in a crowded Dublin restaurant with the band joking back and forth with one another, bringing us into the conversation only from time to time. How could

Stephanie face the frightening ordeal of her upcoming facial and cerebral surgery following such a disappointment? What if the band was not at all as she had envisioned them from their videos? What if she saw them as immature, perhaps even silly as she struggled with realities they could not even comprehend? U2 had become her most powerful link with normal life as her cancer ever so systematically reduced her mobility and erased her senses. And now in a few days, surgery was to take another piece of each and leave her even more visually "different" than she had been in earlier years.

The plane made its slow-motion landing in Shannon for customs clearance, and after a brief stop, it flew at low altitude toward Dublin, a city our family had visited only two years earlier. From twelve thousand feet, there is no greener green than Ireland in May. Green was Stephanie's favorite color, and she loved this sight. With great excitement she reclined her seat, shoved her arm between the two seatbacks, and tapped incessantly on my knee, asking, "Dad, do you see that beautiful green?" I responded that I did but obviously with insufficient gusto to match her need for a more spirited acknowledgment. She repeated twice more, complete with knee tapping, until I said, "Steph, I see it, and it is the most beautiful green I have ever seen." Only then was she satisfied, and she stopped tapping my knee. However, her arm remained poised for more just in case, I suppose, the sight became even more beautiful. I reached forward and held her hand, thankful as I had been since she was eleven weeks old that she could see at all.

CHAPTER 1

Serious, but Not Hopeless

• • •

THE NIGHT OF JANUARY 17, 1968, was clear and dry, allowing a quick return from my evening marketing class at a university about forty miles from our new home in Upstate New York. A few years earlier I would have been inclined to floor the '67 Mustang just to see if it would break a hundred on the county roads. But time and marriage had removed such thoughts from my twenty-eight-year-old mind. My wife was two weeks overdue with our first child, and I wanted to get home safely. We had moved to the United States from Ontario, Canada, eight months earlier and were still getting accustomed to a new life in a new country.

Labor pains began about an hour after I arrived home. A short time later the water broke—an occurrence my naïve mind had previously imagined happening in an orderly and controlled way, not just spontaneously! With that as surprise number one, we made our way in the early morning hours to the local hospital.

Knowing precious little about birth, I expected to see our child in short order. After an extended time, the doctor emerged from behind the swinging doors.

"You may as well go home, because this is going to be a long labor. We'll call you."

Having been raised at a time and in a place where only two types of people had irreproachable knowledge—doctors and teachers—I asked no further questions and went home.

It seemed odd to have received no call by the next morning. However, I dressed and went to work, secure in the knowledge that the doctor would call. About ten o'clock, logic nudged past childhood teachings, and I called the hospital to be told, "You should have been here by now. The baby is on the way." The twenty-minute drive proved too long, and by the time I arrived, we had a daughter.

The experience of first seeing my child was not at all as I had expected. Once again, prior experience—this time movies and books—had let me down. Lying there was not a cooing, smooth-skinned baby with a rattle, but a somewhat jaundiced, terribly tiny being, totally oblivious of me or her surroundings. Her skin was sticky, and her head asymmetrical with a large lump on top. Beginning to panic, I summoned a nurse and inquired as calmly as possible if my daughter would always be like this. With a poorly hidden smile, the nurse responded that the jaundice would soon disappear. Her head, she assured me, would become quite normal, the dislocation having been caused by a long labor. Then she left.

Harboring a lower level of shock and concern, I began to study this tiny baby. Her fingers were so tiny that I wondered at the miracle of their creation. As I studied her, a powerful feeling of amazement and love overcame me. There, in front of me and separate from me, was part of me. A significant level of maturity occurred within me in those few moments.

That night we called the grandparents with the good news. I told my mother that mother and baby—named Tonya at this point—were fine. In all the movies I had seen and all the books I had read, fathers always said, "Fine." The thought of a newborn child not being fine quite simply had never entered my mind. My mother cried and said that she wished my father could be with us to share our joy. My father had died eighteen months earlier from lymphoblastic leukemia, known then as cancer of the blood.

Two days later, a less jaundiced and more symmetrically faced Tonya became Stephanie Anne Lemcke. It seems that we are sometimes able to look at a person and say that she or he is a Gloria or a Vincent instead of a Barbara or a Bob. It was that way with Stephanie. She was not a Tonya. She was clearly Stephanie Anne.

The following morning, on a typically cold Upstate New York January day, we brought her home. Our child-raising years had begun and would progress in logical form—or so we thought. It had been our observation that while handicaps did occur to some people, they were in the province of other families.

Our thoughts were confirmed by the pediatrician after her six-week checkup. "The baby is fine, very healthy," he'd said.

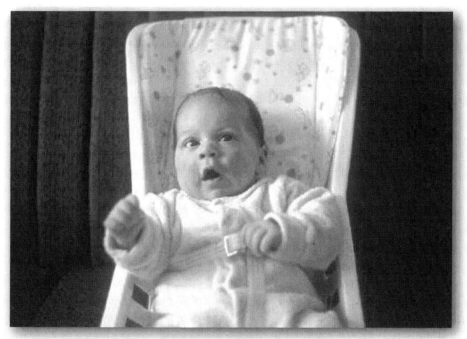

Stephanie at about 6 weeks

In the tenth week of her life, our symmetrically faced, pink-skinned daughter met her second Canadian family. Friends from Toronto had come for the weekend. On the second day of their visit, my friend observed that Stephanie's eyes were moving quickly from side to side. "It looks like they are on an elastic band," I can recall him saying.

A week earlier, I had noticed from across the room what seemed to be a reflection in Stephanie's eye as her mother was feeding her. Comfortable with her six-week checkup, we thought nothing of it. The night our friends left, I again noticed the reflection as I was feeding her. I can recall looking at the ceiling to try to determine what object was appearing as the reflection in her eyes. The combination of the reflection and the eye movement concerned us, so we called the pediatrician the next morning and made an appointment.

Following an examination, the pediatrician immediately referred us to a local ophthalmologist. We became worried when he provided us with the diagnosis that both of her retinas were detached and then told us to visit an ophthalmic specialist in Rochester, New York.

We were not prepared for the words from the Rochester specialist that pierced our ears: "Serious, but not hopeless. I repeat, serious, but not hopeless."

There was a silence in that office—like the silence after a scream in a crowd.

"She has a form of cancer called bilateral retinoblastoma. If it has not spread, it can be controlled. She will have useful but not distinct vision."

"Will she die?" we asked.

"She may. But hopefully it has not metastasized beyond the eyes. If it has not, she should live."

"What is 'useful vision?'" I asked, trying to come to grips with this daytime nightmare.

"She will be able to cook, do housework and broad daily tasks, but she will probably be unable to read or do any activities requiring distinct vision."

As the reality began to sink in, the doctor described this type of cancer. Retinoblastoma ("bilateral" when it occurs in both eyes), he informed us, is a very rare tumor that grows forward rapidly out of the retina toward the front of the eye. As it grows it expands like the cap of a mushroom. In short order the tumor or tumors expand and block light from reaching the retina. As a result, the eye moves from side to side, attempting to position the retina in such a way that it can receive precious light. This mysterious form of cancer occurs both randomly and hereditarily. He advised us that we should take the time to search our family histories for retinoblastoma.

The doctor told us that there was only one place in the world truly qualified to treat Stephanie's cancer—the Eye Institute at Columbia Presbyterian Hospital in New York City.

While the doctor was calling New York, we sat in the waiting room. A lady next to us commented on our beautiful daughter and asked her age. My wife began to cry and hold our baby preciously.

As we approached our car, I suggested for reasons that forever will be unclear to me that rather than holding Stephanie, my wife should put her in the car crib in the backseat. She obviously declined. Years later, I can only conclude that I was somehow trying to prepare for the inevitable— the physical loss of our first child.

As we drove home, Stephanie cooed and played with her rattle, her eyes moving continuously from side to side. We now understood why. At eleven weeks of age Stephanie was totally blind.

Almost nineteen years later we would make that same long drive home from Rochester. "Mother and baby are fine" is not a God-given right.

That night, after Stephanie was asleep, I sat alone struggling with this new reality. A recollection of several dreams or premonitions I had experienced in my early twenties came back to me. Several times during my early working years following college I had dreams of losing a child. I had put them out of my mind as they had no context and made no sense to me. Now those premonitions had a foundation in reality.

Over the weekend, word of Stephanie's cancer spread among our new American friends, and as it did, we experienced the warmth and support so characteristic of this great country. On Sunday night, a friend came to visit and offer support. As we were talking, CBS-TV announced an address by the president of the United States. At its conclusion, Lyndon Johnson put forth an olive branch to the North Vietnamese in an attempt to end that terrible war. He said, "I shall not seek and will not accept the nomination of my party for another term as your president."

"Is that your biggest problem?" I thought.

CHAPTER 2

She'll Live

• • •

OUR APPOINTMENT IN NEW YORK was scheduled for the following Thursday, six days after the diagnosis. Six days is a blink in a lifetime but an eternity when facing the unknown. My attempts to work and our attempts to carry on with the semblance of a normal life at home were, at best, an act.

Retinoblastoma is a particularly opportunistic malignancy, and each night we could see Stephanie's condition worsen. We saw, or thought we saw, her eye begin to bulge, which is a symptom of advanced retinoblastoma. But our options had been set by others. New patients were accepted only on Mondays and Thursdays and on that prior Friday, the following Monday had been booked. In retrospect, I wonder if we should have simply presented ourselves in New York on Monday morning. At least we would have been doing something. Do nothing and you're in for a terrible guilt trip.

Guilt—the gift that keeps on giving.

We flew to Newark, were met by friends, and spent an anxious night awaiting the unfolding of events outside our control. I recall our friends trying to help us take our minds away from our dilemma by playing Scrabble. We could not even come up with words. The next morning we made our way for our first time into that complicated maze called New York City.

In 1968, the Eye Institute was in Columbia Presbyterian Hospital on 168th Street near the Hudson River. It was an oasis of competence and capability in what was an otherwise poor and rundown section of the city. At the hospital, the doctors, nurses, and their assistants were dealing with the thread of life on a day by day basis. At first, we were hurt by their seemingly cavalier attitude as they examined and diagnosed Stephanie. We overhead them joking and engaging in generally light conversation while we, the parents, were agonizing over the outcome of their deliberations. Later, we came to understand. People constantly dealing with death are under tremendous strain. It is actually a blessing that they are able to create a more pleasant work environment to handle the strain. A despondent doctor, as we would experience later, is not a source of strength and confidence.

Following the examination, we met with Dr. Robert Ellsworth, head of the Eye Institute. Having never met him before and knowing literally nothing about him, we felt trapped. Here in front of us was a person—without any credentials we could be sure of—defining our daughter's illness and prescribing her cure. We felt a terrible need to protect her—to somehow be sure that she was in the best hands possible—but we were powerless. It would be some time before we would fully realize our good fortune, or that this would be the beginning of a twenty-year relationship. We would soon learn that Dr. Ellsworth was a pioneer in the research and treatment of retinoblastoma. We were in good hands.

The doctor described clearly and factually what we were facing. And yet he did so with compassion, assuring us that our daughter's condition was not totally hopeless. Dr. Ellsworth was one of those professionals one so rarely meets who has the unique ability to make the candle of eternal hope burn brightly.

"First of all," he said, "she will live."

Then he went on to confirm the diagnosis—bilateral retinoblastoma—perhaps congenital. The treatment procedure had been well established. Her right eye, the one most seriously affected, would be enucleated or, in plain English, removed. This would permit concentrated treatment on her remaining eye in order to shrink the tumors and help Stephanie regain whatever sight might be possible. The postoperative treatment protocol had also been established through years of development. Stephanie would receive regular radiation treatments for a period of five weeks. The total amount of radiation would be the maximum the human skull could accept. Further doses would be extremely risky. This would be our first and last chance to arrest the malignancy, short of removing her second eye. While follow-up chemotherapy was an option, Dr. Ellsworth did not feel her condition warranted that. The operation would occur the following Monday, followed at once by radiation. In the meantime, we were requested to have our eyes examined to begin the process of determining the source of Stephanie's cancer.

Following our sessions, we were brought back to the basic need of finding a place to stay. To our surprise, the answer was right there within the Eye Institute. Dr. Algerman Reese, a co-pioneer of retinoblastoma research, and some of his associates had recognized this need some years before. They had purchased a brownstone house on 165th Street to provide temporary accommodations for the families of children with severe eye disorders. It was not called a Ronald McDonald House because McDonald's had not yet discovered the need, but the concept was firmly in place. It was no four-star hotel, and the tiny elevator constantly threatened to stop, randomly making good on that promise. But at two dollars a day—if you could afford it, and nothing if you could not—it was a godsend. We moved in and began to prepare ourselves for what was to come.

That same day we discovered a second, more substantial advantage of the brownstone: peer support. To our amazement, several other families from many parts of the world were there for the same reason as us. Just having an opportunity to share concerns and exchange ideas about how to cope came as an answered prayer. Within hours of our arrival at the brownstone, we found we were part of a powerful support group.

We had discussions with several families who had been at the Eye Institute for some time, or several times. They seemed to be at ease with the same trauma we were about to face. They were able to assure us that children with this type of cancer do survive. They also gave us early assurance about the high level of expertise we could expect at the hospital.

We also found later about the rare few who are unhealthy company. We were drawn into one discussion about exactly what Stephanie's condition was, and we were given a distinctly negative prognosis based upon the few facts and lots of hearsay. Our solution, as unfair as it may seem, was to simply stay clear of these people. We had the survival of our daughter and our own concerns to cope with, and we decided that was where we would concentrate our energies.

A few years earlier, someone had started a diary at the brownstone for people to write in. We read it and got comfort from reading about children returning for checkups with positive results. A typical entry would read: "Returned for Brian's six-month checkup. The remaining tumor has shrunk and calcified. We do not need to return for one year. God bless Doctors Ellsworth and Reese."

As we studied the diary, we also saw a less optimistic pattern. An entry might read: "Sherry's tumor has still not shrunk. We will be back in two weeks for another checkup." A later entry would read: "Sherry's tumor continues to grow. They will have to enucleate the other eye." And perhaps much later, "The cancer has spread, and we will have to have more treatments." Then, typically, there would be no further entries. It was sobering reading.

I called friends back home. With an unsteady voice I was able to say, "She will live."

Friday morning was set aside for our routine—as we thought—eye examinations and family history review. The family history gave no clues whatsoever, not then, nor later. To anyone's recollection, neither of our families ever had blindness or this type of illness. There is some history of cancer in my family, but it is sporadic. The only activity we felt could have possibly triggered such a development was the set of teeth x-rays my wife had taken during her pregnancy. This was ruled out, however, and the doctors concluded that Stephanie was simply unlucky. We were told that outside the hereditary environment, only one in fifty thousand gets retinoblastoma.

My eye examination followed. After spending too long studying my left eye, Dr. Ellsworth announced that I had a progressive retinal detachment. A detachment is common among physical sports participants, but is normally spontaneous. I had been hit by a softball during a game six years earlier, but for unknown reasons, my detachment had been slowly progressing ever since. I had visited an ophthalmologist months earlier, as I was having some vision problems. However, he found nothing of concern. While it was not dangerously close to traumatic detachment, I was urged to have an operation immediately. "Let's do it," I thought. "Let's get the bad stuff in life behind us all at once."

Events were being prescribed for us. If I wished to maintain vision in both eyes, an operation was mandatory—and very soon. With that, I stayed in New York until Stephanie's operation was performed.

Again, a special procedure had been developed. The doctors removed her eyeball, leaving the muscles intact and wrapping them around a hemispherical piece of plastic. Later, a prosthesis, a plastic eye in the form of a matching hemisphere would fill the eye socket. The prosthesis would move parallel to her normal functioning eye, as the muscles moved it one way or the other. A biopsy of the enucleated eye was performed. The cancer had not metastasized beyond her eyes. We were in a "control" situation. So I could fly to Rochester for my own patch work.

Laser technology was in its infancy in 1968. My retina was therefore reattached through a painful, now outmoded procedure called cryosurgery that required several weeks of convalescence. For four weeks while my wife was in New York with Stephanie, I had my operation and recuperated at home. Finally, after five weeks we were reunited, and I was able to hold my daughter once more. Somehow, she seemed much older. She had lived one third of her short life away from me, and in spite of the treatments, she had grown. She had been fitted with a prosthesis. At the time, we marveled at how natural it appeared. However, looking back at photos years later yields a less positive evaluation. The prosthesis was made much larger than her natural eye in anticipation of skull growth. Her temples were crimson red because of the extensive radiation. But she was home, and we were together.

As I held her, my concentration was on managing each day rather than wondering what the future would bring. There seemed to be so much to deal with in the short term that for then, at least, the long term would have to wait.

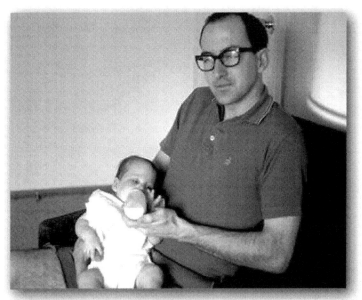

Back home after our operations and her treatments

Over the next several weeks we were extremely anxious about the return of our daughter's vision. The doctors assured us it would happen as the dying tumors gradually receded, permitting light to contact the retina. Far less certain however, was whether the tumors would shrink sufficiently to permit light to make direct contact with the macula, the retina's center. This tiny area the size of a pin head is where distinct vision occurs, where objects have clean edges and sharp colors. Stephanie's ability to read a book or drive a car depended on whether the tumors receded another width of half a pin head. As we waited, I agonized once more over our delay in going to New York after the initial diagnosis. Having watched how quickly the tumors had grown in that short time, the value of each day of earlier treatment was clear to me. I became convinced that if we had simply gone to New York right away without an appointment, Stephanie could have had distinct vision. To this day I carry the burden of that unknown. I vowed during those weeks that if cancer ever came back, we would act swiftly—or, if appropriate—not at all. There would be no in-between.

I have reflected for years on just how much different life could have been for Stephanie if we had acted more quickly on her initial diagnosis.

One may argue that her genes were programmed, so one day here or there would make no difference. That may be true for her overall life, but faster action in those early days may have given her much better sight for the short life she had. A more pragmatic person may very well say what happened is over and cannot be changed, so one should put it out of one's mind. But I cannot, and I have no reason to feel that this burden will not be with me for the rest of my life. I do not look at it as either healthy or unhealthy. It is simply there.

Each morning as Stephanie awoke we would frantically wave our hands in front of her face, hoping for a reaction. One morning she laughed. We were euphoric until we realized from the movement of her hair that her laughter was the result of the air movement caused by our hands passing over her face. We purchased a multicolored wind-up merry-go-round and attached it over her crib. We constantly wound and rewound the toy, waiting desperately for a reaction day after day. One morning about a month after her return home, she responded with a laugh. The same reaction occurred the next day. A few days later, she responded as we stood over her crib. At four-and-one-half months, her sight was coming back. Stephanie would see!

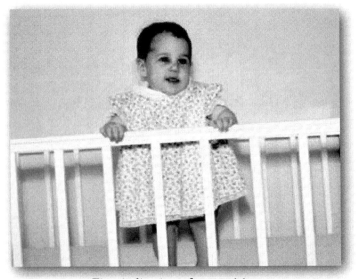

First indication of some vision

CHAPTER 3

Creation of Courage

● ● ●

WITH HER VISION COMING BACK, we felt a level of accomplishment. Once a month for the first half year we returned to the Eye Institute for a checkup. Each time, a blinding light so strong that she cried with pain was shone in Stephanie's eye. Each time the report was the same. Of the three tumors, two were classified as dead and were slowly calcifying—drying up—and turning into a deposit. The one remaining tumor had shrunk and was dormant but still had color. It had not died. At the end of six months, conditions had stabilized and the frequency of visits was reduced to four times per year for the next two years. And the remaining tumor stayed dormant.

The dormant tumor had also shrunk as much as it ever would. It had receded sufficiently for Stephanie to be able to distinguish colors. But it had only receded to the edge of the macula. She would never have distinct vision. Another few dozen microns may have made all the difference. After two years, the checkup frequency was to be reduced to twice yearly, then ultimately once yearly.

The time had come for us to resume normal lives. We had some basic decisions to make about how we should raise Stephanie. Our natural inclination was to be very protective of her. Should anything happen to her remaining eye, we knew she could become totally blind. But as we discussed our options, we realized that there really was only one choice. We would give her all the love in our hearts, but we would raise her with the realization that she would have to survive in a world disinclined to favor or sometimes even accept the handicapped. Stephanie would need to learn that she could never do some everyday things. And she would have to learn and accept that what she could do would often be done with more effort than most others would expend.

We made the same decision on the question of risk. An activity as simple as climbing a tree with its protruding branches would be a risk. We decided to eliminate very few activities and to handle those on an exception basis. That decision paid off in the development of a girl strongly inclined to try rather than to decline. If Stephanie could, we soon found out, she would.

It is difficult to convey the number of decisions we were constantly making or the agony and the joy of practicably applying what was fairly easily decided upon. Judgment calls had to be made every day throughout her development. Could she play in the front yard near the road, or only in the backyard? How much freedom should we give her in playing with other children who would logically not look out for her? Should we let her play with one friendly cat but not another that had a questionable disposition? But establishing a principle at the start and then keeping to it proved invaluable.

We have hundreds of pictures of Stephanie's active childhood, some of which are included in this story. She had a tricycle that she loved to ride. She learned to love the water and became an excellent swimmer. We built snowmen and snow houses in the winter and cut the lawn together in the summer. We did everything a typical family would do. We did it all just a little harder perhaps, with the realization that one day a checkup could show the worst.

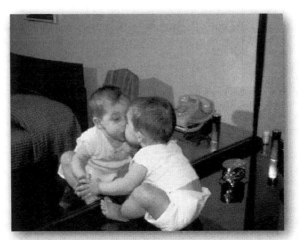

At about 10 months

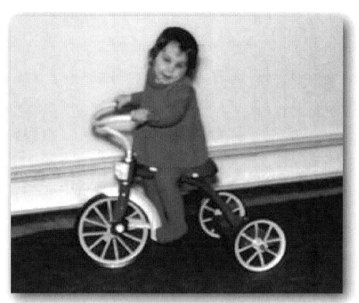

Her first birthday present

To ease her acceptance of her condition at an early age, her prosthesis became her "special eye," so while others had two regular eyes, Stephanie had one regular and one special eye.

Knowing that reading would require extra effort for our daughter, we wanted to establish an early interest in books. So it became a ritual for me to read a book to her each night at bedtime. Years later, I can still recite many books by Dr. Seuss, P. D. Eastman, and others. "Big A little a, what begins with A. Aunt Annie's Alligator. Big B little b, what beings with B. Barber baby bubbles and a bumblebee." And "That Sam I am, that Sam I am, I do not like that Sam I am. Do you like green eggs and ham? Do you like them, Sam I am? Would you eat them on a train? Would you eat them in a plane? I do so like green eggs and ham. I do so like them, Sam I am."

And it worked. The process seemed to stimulate her interest and imagination. She developed her own personal joke. "How do you catch a squirrel? Climb a tree and act like a nut." After laughing so many times at the same joke we felt the need for Stephanie to broaden her repertoire, so we worked on it.

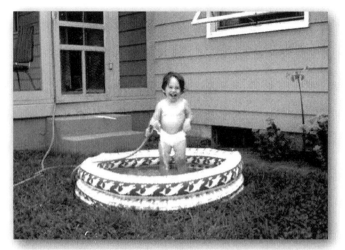

Age about 2

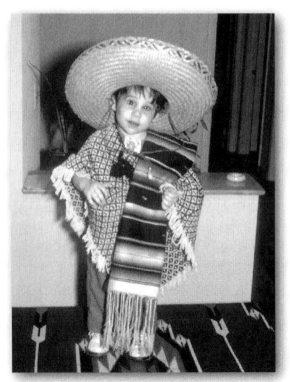

Early signs of character development

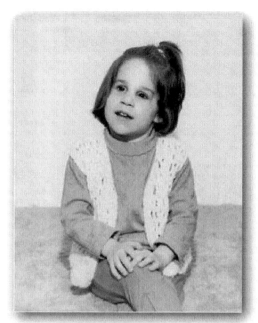

Second birthday

One night when she was two-and-a-half, she asked as the sun was going down, "Does the sun have its blanket when it goes to bed?" During a plane trip to visit our parents the same year, she announced shortly after takeoff and a change in cabin pressure, "Hey, somebody turned me down!"

We bought Stephanie a small, old, wooden school desk. It had a swivel seat and the writing top lifted up, and under that was a storage area for books. This desk became Stephanie's "work area." While others may have been outside learning how to play catch with a ball, Stephanie was "working."

We flooded her with crayons and coloring books and lots of blank pieces of paper. I would often come home from work to find her at her desk, coloring or creating an animal or bird. Since the drawings seldom looked like an animal or a bird I would say, "Stephanie that is pretty; tell me about it." After her description of what it was, I could safely talk about the object. We had purchased an American and Canadian flag for her

(Stephanie carried dual citizenship), and the permanent home for those flags was in the old inkwell on the front of the desk.

And yes, she climbed trees.

As Stephanie developed, we gained a clearer understanding of her potential capabilities and limitations. We had originally planned to have more than one child but had put that decision on hold until we learned more about the amount of attention she would need. We also had to understand more clearly the risk of our second child having retinoblastoma. Having scrupulously checked our family records, we were able to confirm no hereditary traits. So while there was a risk that our second child would have retinoblastoma, that risk was no higher than that of the general population unless, of course, we had missed some family background. With that information we decided that the time had come to have a second child. We felt that Stephanie would be much better off with the love for and support of a sister or brother so we decided to go ahead with a second child.

If we had determined that there was a significant risk in a second child having the disease, we surely would not have gone ahead. We wanted to give Stephanie all the support we could, and it was our feeling that the burden of having two children with such a condition would be unfair to both. In our visits to the Eye Institute, we saw several families of two or more children with this condition. We always wondered why they went ahead and had more children. How could they—parents and children—manage?

By the time Stephanie was aged two-and-a-half or three, we knew she would be able to read large print. But by age four, we felt she would not be able to read regular-size adult print and would need some type of assistance in school. What we did not want for her was a special school for the handicapped.

At the same time, a promise I had made to my wife was coming due. When we moved to the United States in 1967, I promised that once I had gained sufficient industrial experience there, we would return to Canada. That opportunity came in late 1972 with several interviews and a job offer in Toronto that fit well with my business background and objectives.

So with reluctance to leave my excellent current place of employ, I accepted the job and commuted to Toronto during the week for several months. Interspersed were trips to Toronto to find a suitable home. In the midst of spiraling housing costs, we found one in the borough of North York. During our deliberations, we also found to our delight that the city had an excellent program for challenged children. On one such trip, we met with one of the personnel in the special education unit. Her interaction with Stephanie was something to behold. So that one short meeting told us we were in the right place for her also.

On a Sunday evening, I pulled out of our driveway en route to Toronto. Suddenly, after traveling about two miles down the road, I brought the car to a stop on some kind of impulse, turned around, and drove back home. About two hours later, labor pains began and we drove to the hospital. In the early hours of the next morning, with me present, our second daughter was born. In contrast to my first impressions of Stephanie, this seemed to be quite as I'd originally expected. But the emotional impact of seeing my own child was no less the second time around.

Cautious about the potential for retinoblastoma, we had our second daughter examined at birth. A few weeks later, we drove to New York to have her checked at the Eye Institute. There were no signs of retinoblastoma.

The decision about Toronto was even more correct than we could have then imagined. In our efforts to make Stephanie independent, she had developed a level of stubbornness. She was quite reluctant to accept help and had a very determined attitude. At the same time, she had a certain level of reticence born, I am sure, out of a developing realization that she could not do some things very well at all. These traits also may have come out of her early social experiences. As she grew, the effect of the radiation treatment across her temples became more and more noticeable. While the rest of her skull grew normally, this area did not, leaving it indented and somewhat hollow looking. This different appearance began raising innocent questions by her friends at an early age, causing her to be cautious and sometimes withdrawn. While we would do our best to distract other children from staring at her, these efforts were simply ineffective. A child's curiosity is not something that can be controlled at times and not at others.

Stephanie soon learned she could not see what others could. To approximate her level of vision, close one eye and place your fist about four inches in front of your other eye. Your fist represents the dormant tumor. Now concentrate on looking directly at the center of your fist, and at the same time select an object on the periphery of the fist. You will notice that you can see the color of the object, but you will not be able to see the details of its features. Objects immediately beyond your fist are not visible to you at all. To see them, move your eye inward toward your nose, and move your fist with it, always looking at the center of your fist. Now you can see what was beyond your fist but, as before, the object is not distinct. This is what and how Stephanie saw. In order to get a full picture of an object, she would move her eye from side to side, remembering what was in the last area of vision. With a few side to side eye movements, she would literally piece together an image of the objects in front of her. No lens, no operation, no technology available then (or now, to the best of my knowledge) could help her see any better.

Stephanie also discovered at about age five that she could stimulate her sight by pushing in on her eye with her finger. The potential for her doing damage caused us concern, but the doctors who were familiar with the habit assured us this would not happen. Apparently, this action serves to stimulate the retina, assisting in forming images.

Between pushing in on her eye and rotating it from side to side, she drew even more attention. As the years progressed, this habit would elicit cutting, cruel remarks from her peers. So her barriers of protection ascended at an early age. She needed constant reaffirmation to maintain her sense of self-esteem.

We spent a lot of time creating the environment for her to reach that sense. We constantly gave her positive reinforcement and encouraged her to try in spite of difficulties. But that was often not enough to overcome her feelings. Too often others in a crowd would stare right at her and then make a whispering comment to a friend followed by a snicker as they walked off. Stephanie would sometimes say, "Let's go home now." I recall once while we were shopping, Stephanie leaned forward to more clearly see a toy horse on a shelf. She did not see an adjacent protruding hook, which hit her right in the middle of her prosthesis as she leaned forward. I could see the humiliation on her face as she stepped back. It was only after much coaxing that she more carefully studied the toy. But the joy of the moment was gone.

The special education group of North York school system in Toronto knew all of this and was equipped to help us handle it. They determined that her vision was 20/400. That is, she could see at twenty feet what others could see at four hundred. They knew better than we the level of frustration she was to face and how to help her release that. In spite of her poor vision, they agreed that Stephanie had enough sight, even though 20/200 is defined as legally blind, to mainstream in a regular school system rather than attend a school for the blind. I do not know what our reaction would have been if they had decided otherwise.

The special education group worked as a support system for the regular school. Teachers were given training as to what to expect from the challenged and why. They were provided various types of visual aids for assistance. Large print books were available. And most schools had a resource room that was reserved for the special education advisor assigned to work privately with the child during visits to the school. It was also a place where the child, in the presence of the advisor, could diffuse his or her built-up frustrations. After sessions with the child, the advisor then provided feedback to the teacher, advising where changes in approach were needed. The system had its shortcomings, borne out of lack of time, pride, ego, stubbornness, and whatever other characteristics keep the human race removed from the elusive goal of perfection. But it worked, and usually well. And, for Stephanie, it worked very well.

Many have experienced the tremendous impact of a mentor. Such was the case with Stephanie. The first person she met in the Toronto education system and the one that made our return to Toronto so meaningful was Miss Jean Mills in the Special Education Unit of the North York school system. Miss Mills seemed to have the ability to guide Stephanie like no one else we'd met before or since. In their first meeting, Miss Mills asked Stephanie to assemble some blocks as a test of her vision and eye-hand coordination. Stephanie, probably sensing one more doctor-type test, refused. Miss Mills immediately coaxed her in a gentle way, and to our amazement, Stephanie quickly did exactly what Miss Mills wanted. And Stephanie loved her. For most of her Toronto education, Miss Mills was her counselor. So Miss Mills, wherever you are, God bless you.

But that system would prove to be only a part of what she would need. We found, starting from a very early age, she needed constant support at home. Perhaps we taught her too well that she would have to exert more effort than others to achieve, as her personal goal from the early days of kindergarten was to stay with the pack. To achieve this she often stayed after school and constantly brought her work home. Her mother became her second teacher. Each night, they would work together—a short time at first—extending to literally all evening in later years. And at home, perhaps more than at school, Stephanie would vent her frustrations. She would often say, "I'm not going to do anymore!" But invariably, with a little coaxing, she would return to her books and finish her assignments.

We did not want Stephanie to have to cross a road on her way to school, so we chose a house in North York that backed up on the playground of the school we had chosen. Soon after starting at the school, we discovered that it operated under the "open" concept, an experimental system wherein students were permitted a high degree of freedom to do literally as they wished. Within a few months, it became clear that this was not the environment for a child in need of constant attention. So at the conclusion of kindergarten, Stephanie was transferred to a conventional learning school a few blocks away. Her mother or a friend drove or walked with her to and from school each day.

Stephanie became active in music and after-school art and social activities programs. On one occasion at the new school, her supplementary activity was canceled and she decided to walk home. She soon became lost.

Later, a teacher at school found her outside, crying. She called her mother who came to rescue her. When asked how she was able to return to the school, Stephanie proudly announced that she had retraced her footsteps in the snow.

Music was difficult for Stephanie, but she stayed with it. She was unable to read regular music print, so her mother transcribed each score into a larger size, permitting Stephanie to read. She loved her music, and we bought a piano for her. Later, she would play the flute, an instrument she stayed with throughout high school.

And she had her own learning experiences that helped her to decide her limits for herself. During our first year in Toronto, we decided to purchase a two-wheeler for her. Our instructions were clear: "Do not go off the sidewalk, and do not go across the road. If you come to a driveway, you must look toward the road three times to be sure there is no car coming." And she would do it. We would watch her sharply turn her head toward the road one, two, and then three times. But limits of speed were learned the hard way during her first ride on the two-wheeler. It had training wheels and was bright green in color (green had become her favorite color outdistancing all others to the point that there was no contest. When asked what her favorite color was, "*Green!*" came back with the speed of a bullet). As she rode her new green two-wheeler down the sidewalk way too fast, she came upon a hill. Down she went even faster until the inevitable happened, and she took a bad spill. I wanted to rush down the street, pick her up, and hold her. Her mother, with a greater level of calm, correctly said, "She must handle it herself." She did, and returned, bruised physically and emotionally but without tears.

In kindergarten, she enrolled in ballet and conventional dance classes. Whereas others could easily follow the instructor's dance steps, she had difficulty as she could simply not see well enough. To accommodate, she would look both at the teacher in front of her and the other students to her side. We have photos of her in ballet. While others are looking straight ahead, Stephanie's head is turned to the side, following the others. She continued in ballet until she was nine and thereafter switched to jazz tap dancing, which she studied for several years.

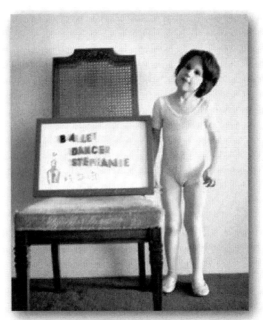

Kindergarten Ballet

Her fine artistic ability, if hereditarily assumed, clearly did not come from her father, but the other side of the family. Whether from genes or external environment, that ability that had begun in the work area school desk at home blossomed in kindergarten. Drawings she made of the family always had smiling faces. Sometimes one of the four in the picture had only one eye. As kindergarten progressed, she began drawing horses, and they would remain a special love her whole life. Her kindergarten graduating report card read as follows:

Stephanie is socially and emotionally alert and conscientious. She readily participates in activities and plays well with other children. She is able to work well without supervision. Her physical overall coordination is good. Academically, she knows the alphabet and recognizes consonants. She knows many rhyming words, speaks in complete sentences, and has an above-average vocabulary. She knows the colors and recognizes and prints her name. She matches patterns from left to right. She recognizes numbers to ten, counts objects, and recognizes basic geometric shapes. Paintings, drawings, and hand work are well above average. Paintings show good detail and thought. Good luck in grade one.

This was a substantial improvement from her midyear report, which had read:

Catching balls—does her best
Emotional—gaining confidence
Mathematics—refuses to count to twenty

After Stephanie completed kindergarten, we decided to rent a cottage on beautiful Lake Simcoe, north of Toronto, for our summer vacation. We found ourselves in the midst of horse country, surrounded by horse shows. We knew of Stephanie's interest and decided to take her for a horse ride. The horse was called Emmagee, and Stephanie was immediately attracted to her. As she was lifted onto the saddle, she said, "I want to steer it!" And steer it she did. Little did we know the overwhelming impact that would result from choosing our 1974 vacation in horse country.

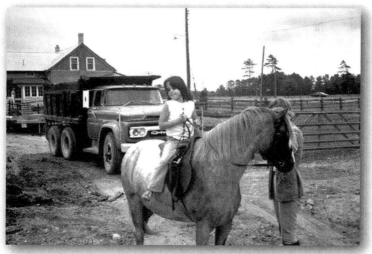

With Emagee – I want to steer it

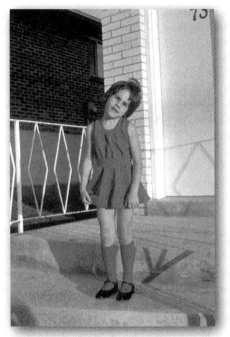

First day – Grade I

The pattern of her development became more clear in grade one. She continued with ballet and began piano lessons. Written communications became important to her and as it did, we could see the beginning of her difficulty with spelling. Perhaps because she couldn't see a complete word, she had great problems. Wanting to use my calculator, she wrote the following:

Ples can I eus your ading mishyn. I wil giv you a presint.

At school, she wrote a poem:

My Horse, by Stephanie
I wich I wrr a horse
I'd eat and dringck
I'd tak you for a rid Win I
like you I'd tak you too
        The end

We had decided that a skateboard with its sensitive steering system was too risky for her. She wrote, "A skatboard is a board with two skats on the bottom. I am knot alowd to have one because I mit tip over."

At the conclusion of grade one, her report card read:

> *Stephanie is a quiet, conscientious girl who has made steady progress. She is hesitant to answer oral questions, but does quite well on written assignments. Her news stories are interesting. Her pictures are quite detailed and mature. She really enjoys music. She has made satisfactory progress in math. Stephanie works slowly but steadily and accepts responsibility.*

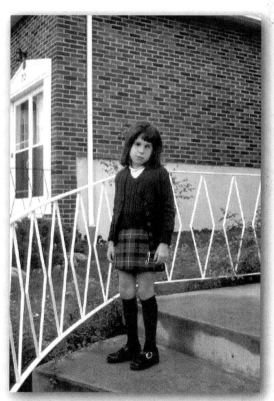

First day – Grade II

At the conclusion of grade two, she was rated at the expected level with "great ideas, well expressed" written in the comment section on her stories. Her teacher wrote:

Stephanie has made nice progress. Her reading has improved with practice. She is able to identify all words, but at a slow rate. Stephanie has caught on to the new concept of multiplication. She has participated more this term and has become a more outgoing member of the class. Promoted to grade three. Best of luck, Steph!

As her abilities at school developed, we continued to hope that her vision would improve. And we thought from time to time that it was. Our phone was a rotary-dial type, typical for that era. As she began to use the instrument, she was unable to see the numbers. To dial, she would move her first and second fingers, like walking from one hole to the next, counting until she reached the number she wanted. Rotating the dial and letting it return, she would go on to the next in the same fashion until all numbers had been dialed. Later, she was able to complete the process much more rapidly. Our thought, or perhaps hope, was that her vision was improving. What we should have accepted was that her other senses were progressively making up for her lack of vision.

One day in the third grade, Stephanie complained that she was seeing spots. We immediately made an appointment to visit the Eye Institute in New York. To our relief, the doctors saw no change. However, having gone through that experience, I felt a terrible need to know more about what may lie ahead of us. So I wrote to Dr. Ellsworth, asking about the statistics and the potential for a return of cancer. His response came to us a week later. In as positive a way as possible yet with honesty, the doctor told us what we perhaps would have been better off not knowing. Yes, he responded, there is a history of a recurrence of cancer in retinoblastoma patients. He did not give statistics. From our later research, I think that knowing the full story then would not have been positive for us as a family. Statistics show quite clearly that in the second decade following treatment for retinoblastoma, a recurrence of cancer is highly probable, often appearing as a sarcoma in the leg opposite the most affected eye.

CHAPTER 4

The Cruelty of Adolescence

● ● ●

It was clear to us during her third grade that the North York system had done wonders for Stephanie. Although she was finding it more difficult to read the progressively smaller print, she was coping well.

At the same time, my frustration level was growing. I had enjoyed excellent career development in the United States. Now, back in Canada, while I had a very good job, I felt out of the stream of action compared to the faster pace of American business. After starting my career in Canada, I had made a fortunate shift at age twenty-five to a position that allowed us to move to the United States two years later. Having watched my Canadian boss constantly making phone calls to the American parent for decisions that I felt should be under our local control, I decided that while I was certainly in the right business, I was in the wrong country. (I coined the term "truncated management" to characterize the fact that one could enjoy a certain amount of growth in Canada, but beyond a point, one's career development was cut off due to the fact that most companies were foreign owned and the shots were being called elsewhere.) Now back in Canada, I found much to my surprise that I had become quite Americanized. I found it difficult to assimilate back into the more conservative Canadian culture prevalent in this industry.

Shortly after our return to Canada, while I still had New York State license plates on my car, we attended a Toronto football game. On exiting the stadium, youths pounded on the car shouting, "Go home, Yankee!" I rolled down my window and shouted that I was a Canadian, back home, doing more for the country than they were. At that moment I felt no part a Canadian and said, "We're moving back to the States." Later that evening, I became calmer.

In the fall of 1977, I received a job offer I felt I could not turn down. A senior sales and marketing management position with a large, American-based, highly international corporation was more than I could say no to. I accepted. While we did discuss Stephanie's needs, I am not at all sure I gave them full attention. More guilt, here we come.

We decided that the family would continue to live in Toronto until near the end of the school year. After receiving grades, we would move to New Jersey so Stephanie could attend the last few weeks of school in our new home. After a session with the superintendent of schools, school principals, and guidance counselors, we chose the beautiful suburban New Jersey community of Summit, nestled in the Watchung Hills. To our pleasure, we found that this school system had a support group for the handicapped. It did not compare to Toronto, but it was in place and ready to help.

As an introduction to Stephanie, her principal in Toronto provided the following letter:

I am writing on behalf of Stephanie Lemcke about whom I am sure some specific information will be of help. She is a very interesting child who has a great strength of character. In general, Stephanie's academic progress has been steady at the grade three level. While she demonstrates above average ability in her reading comprehension, vocabulary, and creative writing, she works extremely slowly. Work she cannot complete she insists on taking home.

She works best with a maximum of individual direction and help. Group work tends to add too much confusion. In both large and small group instruction she tends to tune out a little and requires individual assistance afterward.

Obviously Stephanie's limited vision calls for sensitivity and an adjusted teaching methodology. She requires a reasonable amount of direct reinforcement for jobs well done and understanding on days when her patience is frayed. We have found her to be a fairly open, talkative, and extremely affectionate little girl as soon as her surroundings are familiar to her.

In mathematics the class has been studying the metric system. Stephanie has a fairly good basic understanding of length, mass, and capacity in metric measure. Her knowledge of the Imperial System may be limited. In general, her work in math is at level.

I hope this short introduction will be of some help. We hope that Stephanie's plucky manner will continue to carry her through. Her parents are incredibly understanding and helpful. I wish them all the very best.

Our life in New Jersey began beautifully. Stephanie made friends early. We spent Easter break working on our new home. A neighbor of Stephanie's age came over, and the two of them went to play by a brook that bubbled its way through our wooded backyard. Sometime later when they separated, Stephanie announced, "Well, you can consider her my first friend."

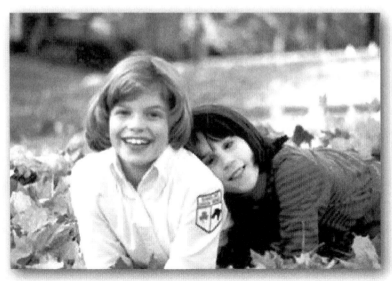

Hallie – her first New Jersey friend

Shortly after we moved in, the Tighlman family with four children both older and younger than ours moved in next door. We almost immediately became friends. This was a friendship without age stratification. Everyone was a friend of everyone. Their youngest, aged two, and I had long discussions. The same was true with the others. The kids would play alternatively with one and then the other without territorial proclamations or disagreements. Their oldest, Jenny, and Stephanie decided they needed a special secret communication device. So we purchased two pulleys, some rope, and set up the equivalent of a moveable clothesline above our driveway and between their bedrooms. They would write their secret messages, reel them across, and then read them aloud to each other.

The Tighlmans erected a device they called a space trolley between two trees in their backyard. It was again strung like a clothesline but complete with a carrier on pulleys that would, after a push, carry a person from one tree to the other. The kids played on that trolley until the grass below realized there was nothing to be gained by attempting to raise even a blade.

Halloween became a ritual during our New Jersey years. Occasions such as this were becoming major benchmarks in Stephanie's life, and a custom-designed outfit was crucial. One year her mother made a bumblebee costume, and Stephanie stole the show. It was a cold night as I recall, but Stephanie was giving such delight at each door that we went on and on. At each door I would say, "Just one more, Steph," and she would respond, "OK, Dad, but only one."

Swimming became even more important, perhaps as a release for her frustration. Both Stephanie and her sister loved swimming. As a result, the Summit community pool became a common ground for us and our neighbors.

During our first summer, we discovered a riding stable within the city. We enrolled Stephanie and literally from her first Saturday, those weekly lessons became the focal point of her life. Each Saturday morning she would dress in English riding attire, and we would rush to the stables. She would fearlessly mingle among the horses, each fully twice her height, and somehow find her assigned horse. She would then mount up, make her way into the ring, and take her lesson from the barking instructor, the way it seems to be done in English saddle. She became very good very quickly and soon won her first ribbon. In the photograph we took of her following her successful competition, one can see a dot of a child sitting on an over-sized horse. A closer view reveals a somewhat concealed, one-sided smile of accomplishment.

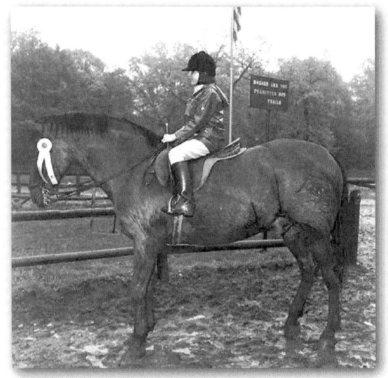

Her first ribbon

Later, at school, she would write a story called "My Dream":

I dreamed I was at a horse selling stable, and I saw a horse I liked. It cost three thousand dollars and I brought two thousand dollars. I asked the lady if I could buy it for two thousand dollars. She said yes because the price had changed. I took the horse home and built a stable for it. Then I went to bed.

The next year, she wrote, "My Wish":

> I wish I owned a field a mile long and a mile wide with one hundred horses inside. It would have the greenest grass and a white fence around it. The horses would be the best breads [her spelling, while greatly improved, lacked perfection] and the best colors.
>
> There would be the best water in a pond, ner the middle. In the ring there wold be rocks and trees for the horses to feel at home. I would live in a mantion at the edge of the field and help the horses if they had a problem.

The first year in New Jersey also taught our children the fragility of life and the reality of death. While still in Toronto, we'd bought a cat for Stephanie. She attempted to select its name from among three—Peanuts, Tab, and Marbles. Unable to select, she kept all three and the cat became PTM. For reasons known only to PTM, it elected one day to sleep on the engine of my car. I entered and started the engine. A groan from the engine was the only clue I received that something was not right. Backing away, I saw PTM dead on the drive, obviously having made its way through the fan or fan belt. Fortunately, there was no external evidence of trauma. My wife brought the children out, and they held the remains of our family member. They then proceeded to bury it in the backyard. Stephanie was very quiet, very circumspect. If she did cry, it was not in front of us.

Recovery from the loss was important. We quickly found another cat. The cat was black, so the name branding exercise was simpler. It became Licorice—or, in Stephanie's phonetic spelling Likorish. As a way of offsetting her grief we also bought her a bird. On a Saturday morning, Stephanie and I went to a local pet store to choose the bird and accessories. The choice was rapid—a parakeet—green, of course. It became Julep and lived happily with us for years.

As we knew it would, the print in the grade four books became markedly smaller. We purchased a magnifying glass, which Stephanie agreed to use at home but not at school. Each night, she would struggle with her homework, her nose against the magnifying glass as her hand coaxed it across each page. Large-print books were available, but she strongly re-sisted using them, particularly at school. At home, she would use talking books, which were available for some courses. As she approached adoles-cence, she wanted very much to be like everyone else. She insisted on completing her assignments and her mother tirelessly helped her, often too late into the evening, past the bedtime for a child of ten.

For Stephanie to see, copied sheets had to be clear. But the copied material from school was often terribly hard to read. It became neces-sary for us to meet regularly with the teachers to explain her needs. We finally discovered that it helped to place a yellow transparency sheet over the copied pages, so this became a standard part of her school supplies. In later years, friends would take notes in class, and we would have them copied for Stephanie. She was unable to follow the class and keep notes at the same time. Writing was simply too consuming.

Still, she loved to write and paint. In grade four she put together her own book. The cover stated: "My Drawing Book by Stephanie Lemcke."

There are lots of things in this book
So open it up and take a look.

Inside was her family "Coat of Arms." It was a beautiful piece of work, using paper, cloth, cotton batting, and other materials in various shapes, coming right out of the page.

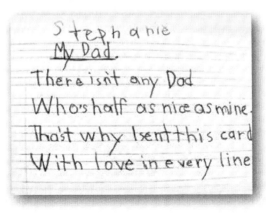

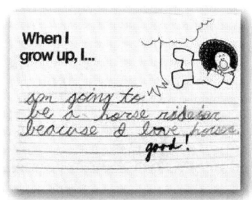

When I
grow up, I...

am going to be a horse rider because I love horses.

Some spelling work required

As she entered the adolescent years, the pain of being different became a very difficult experience. While others knew she looked and acted differently, the excellent fittings she had been given provided no clue that she had a plastic eye. She was due for a new fitting and innocently told classmates she was going into New York the next day for a new special eye. The result was devastating. She became "Cyclops" to her classmates. They would chase her home and taunt her. Some would even telephone her at home and shout "Cyclops!"

One day when returning home in the rain, someone threw stones at her, hitting her umbrella. That experience traumatized her for a long time. But in spite of it, her report cards for her three school years at Lincoln show her being tardy only twice. Toward the end of her life, her mother asked her what had been her most difficult experience. She quickly responded, "The kids at Lincoln School."

From her first grade, we had always arranged for her to sit in the front row to help her see the chalkboard. This bothered her, and she often asked why she was made to sit in the front. We also encouraged her to get up and go to the board to read when she could not see. In her early school years, she did this. But as time went on and she was teased, she refused.

Upon entering her fifth grade, one of her teachers sat her in the middle of the room in spite of our preparatory meetings. Stephanie did not ask to be seated at the front, probably delighted to be more like the others.

After a week we discovered the error and she moved up, disappointed, but knowing this was how it must be.

Loyal friends were few during those adolescent years. She could count on Hallie, her friend across the street, the Tighlman kids next door, and Christine who lived nearby. They would play together after school, and from time to time one of them would go to riding classes and watch Stephanie. And as time passed and the harassment and teasing she was subjected to continued, we saw significant transformations in her. The first was inevitable. She became far more cautious about initiating contact, less positive about making new friends, and much more careful about preserving secure relationships. She wrote a note in grade six:

> *Dear Hallie,*
>   *I am sorry for teasing you about Chris. I didn't mean to make you made at me. Put this noat and little picture with something on the back in your noat box.*
>   *Love*
>   *Steph*

As was becoming her custom, whether on notes or schoolwork assignments, a drawing of an animal, this time a mouse, appeared beside her name.

As she came to expect less from the outside world, her energies turned more toward things she could influence and her focus sharpened. Christmas became very important, and the planning and list-making seemed to begin even before the shops in the malls initiated their rush toward the pocketbooks of New Jersey. She tended toward making rather than buying gifts and cards. She took countless hours to make me a holder for nails and screws. She saved small jars and nailed the tops to a long, square piece of wood she'd found. Each end received a nail for suspension, and a long wire communicated between them. The whole apparatus was designed to rotate, providing easy access for my supplies. (A second objective, I suspect, was subtle suggestion to make my workshop tidier.)

Tree decoration was an important event, and she made special tree ornaments. When the time to decorate approached, Stephanie seemed to take the lead. In grade five at school, she elected to write a story about a Christmas tree and subsequently placed it in a bright green cover, complete with her artistic interpretation of the tree:

"The Adventures of a Christmas Tree Forest to Home"

Once there was a Christmas tree named Kerry.

One day Kerry saw some peopole walking in the forest, they were coming closer to her.

The family came closer. When they got to the trunk she felt lik screaming because it hurt so much when the man hit her with the ax

After that, they took her from the forest to they're home.

It was a weird ride home, she had never seen cars or been in the trunk of one before.

When they got home, they set her in a pot of lots of water. They wanted to give her lots of water, because they knew the next day was Christmas. Then they put presents under Kerry.

The next day Kerry was wakened by the breakfast dishes clacking in the kitchen, and a man came out and watered her.

He called everybody. They came out with decorations, they started to decorate Kerry.

After they finished decorating her, they put more presents under Kerry.

That Kerry was wakened by a Ho-Ho-Ho! She opened her eyes and saw a little fat man, she thought it was Santa Claus. It was. She saw the S.C. on his belt.

In the morning everybody took the candies and choclets S.C. left on the tree. Then everybody opend presentes.

The next day they had to put Kerry in the garage and clean up her needles.

She developed a story for literature class called "Rats on Cats." The cover drawing shows in great detail a picture of a rat riding on a cat. A bunny is running by, its fur actually colored cotton balls. The clouds are white cotton balls stuck with glue onto the heavy front cover. Excerpts from the study inside go like this:

> No cats in Cratsvill would dare to go neer Von Graycat because they knew he had the longest whip in Cratsvill. When any hungry cat got as far as three feet away from him, he would take out his whip and hit them so hard, that they would run to Pittsburgh wich was 40 miles away, without stopping.
>
> Von Graycat was also the best cat rider and the best in the Catsvill Rodeo.

The eight-page story is intertwined with three full pages of watercolors. Other characters develop in the story, including a Persian cat named Snowpuff, concluding with Von Graycat and Sheriff Bill getting their names in the newspaper and an award of appreciation from the mayor of Cratsvill, all for getting the cats out of Pittsburgh. She got an A.

A neighbor across the street was a retired executive who painted and made ceramic birds as a hobby. His creativity was so impressive he surely could have made his living in art had he so desired. He became aware of Stephanie's abilities through a sketch Stephanie had given his wife as a gift at Christmas. He asked if we would let him teach her art. We agreed.

Once or twice each week after school, Stephanie would make her way to Mr. Soward's house for her art lesson. His creativity was exceeded only by his abruptness, and at first this required some accommodation by Stephanie. In fact, Mr. Soward may have been the seed for the development of her ability to reduce thoughts to their lowest common denominator in a few words or phrases. As years passed, she developed an acute knack to be clearly understood with a few well-chosen words when the situation warranted it.

Her ability in art took a great leap forward from those lessons. She was taught the bone structure of animals as part of the preparation. And from there she learned the importance of perspective. As her ability developed, she began to draw birds and various types of animals, often horses. In all, it was a great experience.

From time to time, Mr. Soward and I visited to discuss the world, the Dow Jones Industrial Index, and the price of gold. On one of our visits he exclaimed, "Let me tell you one damned thing—that kid's got it."

Through the handicapped support system, we discovered a summer camp—Camp Marcella, near Hepatcong, New Jersey. The camp was run by the State Commission for the Blind. Stephanie expressed an interest, so we enrolled her during our second summer.

At Camp Marcella, Stephanie was playing on a level field. She had an opportunity to make friends with true peers. And here she was able to understand there were others less fortunate than she. Through this experience, she was able to return from camp more prepared to go on in the unfriendly world of adolescence.

Every attendee at Camp Marcella won at least one award. Stephanie won awards for swimming and running. The last summer she attended the camp, we became progressively more concerned during the closing ceremony as awards were presented for events we had expected her to win. As my heart sank, I could see her there in front of us, her shoulders slumping just a little more as each name was called. I almost went up to one of her counselors to explain their omission before it was too late. In the middle of that contemplation, the final award was announced, and I almost panicked that I had waited too long. The award was to be given to the most valued participant at Camp Marcella. Following several accolades for excellence in sports, leadership, and character, the name Stephanie Lemcke was called. In her quiet way, she stepped forth to accept. Tears came to my eyes.

Following that experience, Stephanie entered the sixth grade track meet. Literally, without practice, she won the school championship—one-half mile at 3:57.

But even in her fifth grade, we were concluding that the Summit school system, in the long pull, would prove to be too much for her to handle. New Jersey, like much of the metropolitan New York area, is a high-achievement culture. Many parents are executives and expect results from their children. The school system is designed to satisfy these parental ambitions, and the money is there to support them. While this environment proved no problem for her sister, it certainly placed a heavy load on Stephanie.

But she was working at grade level. In grade four, she achieved three As and three Bs. Her report card read, "Steph continues to improve and put forth great effort." In grade five, she got two As, three Bs and a C. The teachers' comments were flowery. November 6, 1978: "Stephanie is a very hard working student. It's a pleasure to have her." February 12, 1979: "Stephanie is a very talented and creative young lady." April 9, 1979: "Stephanie has an amazing capacity to overcome frustration. Her test grades slumped a bit in Social Studies. Her report, however, was outstanding." June 19, 1979: "There continues to be a very super effort by Stephanie to do her best." In grade six, she would achieve one A, three Bs and two Cs. The operative word throughout her reports was "effort." But we asked ourselves, when was more and more effort born from desire to be just like the others too much?

We pondered what to do. There was a school for the blind in Morristown, about thirty miles away—too far for a daily commute. Moreover, we did not feel in our hearts that this was a good option for Stephanie. Her mother had meetings with private schools in the area and ascertained that these schools were targeted at the high-achievement sector of the population. We did not know what to do next.

In the spring of 1979, I received a call from a man who had for years been my business mentor. Following a sabbatical from the company he and I had worked for in Upstate New York State years earlier, he had recently returned as president. "Why don't we talk?" he asked. It all seemed to come together. The job was right for my career. The area was more rural and far less pressure-oriented, which would be advantageous for Stephanie. The school system, we knew, did not measure up to New Jersey's, and that would be less advantageous for her sister. So we reached our conclusion. We would move back to Upstate New York.

CHAPTER 5

Coming Home, in Many Ways

● ● ●

STEPHANIE WAS DISTURBED AND DISAPPOINTED. "You promised we would not move again. You promised."

I had, and she wanted to be sure I knew it. I developed a deep feeling of guilt. Two of the clear teachings I'd received as a child were honesty and fulfillment of a commitment. I had broken my own code.

Stephanie needed and wanted consistency of her surroundings. We stayed in New Jersey for one year following my acceptance of the new job. But now I would transfer to corporate headquarters in Upstate New York. While we were sure it would be better for Stephanie, she had no reason to share that belief.

Stephanie always had fine friends—loyal and understanding—who saw beyond her different appearance. She greatly valued those relationships. One of her best friends was a schoolmate named Nga who had escaped with her family from Vietnam in a boat, giving up their possessions and crossing the South China Sea to freedom. They had arrived in New Jersey and were in the process of building a new life. Sacrifice was common to Stephanie and Nga, and it was this element that created the bond.

We struck a compromise. We would buy Stephanie a horse as soon as we relocated. We had always been uneasy about her riding, fearing an accident. In the end, our earlier decision about risk prevailed. Stephanie would have her horse. (And she would keep her old friends. She never stopped corresponding with Nga, for example.)

As we had done in our move from Toronto, the children and their mother stayed in New Jersey to the end of the school year. We then moved up, first to a rented home and then to our permanent residence. Stephanie did not immediately fall in love with our purchased home. She called it "our mausoleum."

In September, Stephanie began grade seven. We settled in for what we expected to be the rest of our lives. For the wrong reasons, we were partly right.

The cruelty of adolescence, we found, did not have territorial boundaries. As seems to exist everywhere in the world, smaller, more rural communities have a friendlier atmosphere—a certain bonding more difficult to find in metropolitan areas. While this smaller community was much kinder, the basic problems still existed.

At school, she experienced the same treatment. Some classmates constantly raided her locker, teased her at gym classes for her obvious inability to participate in various sports, and generally harassed her at lunch. She wrote in a diary:

> *Today somebody got my lunch again. With a striped bag too. I'm going to make a catfood sandwich sooner or later!*

She maintained active participation in the school band and played in all the concerts. Sitting at the back of the auditorium, we felt sorry and helpless watching her sit down at the front among the group as they waited for their turn, only to witness the others form into groups away from her, leaving her sitting quite alone. As a result, she often felt self-conscious. She wrote in a grade nine journal:

> *Today in Spanish Suzy told me my shirt was inside out. So I changed it and it's all scuzzy. I swear, the worst things happen to me!*

But as time progressed, she learned how to manage this adversity, and the adversity itself also began to fade. She developed friendships with those we had kept in touch with from our first stay in the area, and she also made a few key friends who would stand by her. She wrote in her diary:

Maya keeps making me eat lunch with her in the band hall. She says I'm fun to be with. Marya and I played tennis today. I couldn't hit 'em back too well.

By grade nine, the social scene was improving for her, and her interest in boys made its sudden—if not unexpected—appearance. She developed a crush on a senior who worked in a drugstore downtown, and our needs for household products from that store seemed to suddenly explode. One of her friends gave him the nickname "Fish." She wrote:

Karen keeps calling me "Fish" down the hall. Now she's found the French word for fish. Before she called me French Fish. I still don't think he looks like a fish. I hope he doesn't find out about this fishy business.

And later:

Karen called me Superfish in the hall. So did Marya. I give up!

Ultimately, she became "Womanfish," and one of the many signs on her bedroom door was "Womanfish's Room."

But true boyfriends eluded her. At fifteen, boys were no doubt looking for the cute, popular girls. At age fifteen, she wrote in her school journal:

There's another dance this Friday. I'm not going again. Nobody can stand me yet. Last time when I didn't come, they called me and asked me to come anyway.

But she was invited to that dance by a teenage family friend. Either through a yet-to-be-developed sense of social etiquette or impatience, she walked to the dance at the appointed time. When her date came by to pick her up, slightly late, we had to explain that Stephanie had already left. After that dance, she wrote about another classmate:

> *Bill asked me to dance with him. There's no way he's going to make up for all that crap he used to do to me. Throwing cookies—call me autistic—throwing more cookies, etc. I skipped lunch before because of him. And there he was, asking me if I'd like to dance with him!*

Othello is a complicated board game where the idea is to comprehend not what is there on the board in front of you, but rather what could be there. In spite of her limited vision, Stephanie excelled at this game. When I first taught her, I made sure I lost at least half of the time. After a few games, I tried my best and was able to win perhaps one out of three. She wrote:

> *Sue slept over the other night and we painted my bathroom. Then we played Othello. And, of course, we listened to the stereo.*

We had to deal with the concept of earning power with Stephanie. Because of her condition, she could not expect to get a "regular" job. She did baby-sit twice for people who understood her competence and commitment. However, her only logical source of income was her weekly allowance. From this, she diligently saved for her first stereo. Later, when she contracted cancer, we became less inclined to teach her the rules of financial responsibility, and we would try to give her whatever we could without spoiling her.

The sixteenth birthday is a watershed in many ways—in New York, it is legal driving age. Two entries in her journal read:

> *Next weekend I get to have sixteen chicks sleep over! My birthday is the eighteenth. I'm so mad I not gunna get to drive!!*

And later:

> *I need to make cookies for Miss Lott. Her birthday was the 14th. Mine is the 18th and I'll be sixteen. I wish I could drive. Oh well, I'll be a taxi woman.*

Through it all, she developed some definitive likes and dislikes. She articulated these in her grade nine journal:

Most Liked	Hated
Rock Concerts	School
Food	Traveling
The Pets	Cruddy music
Horse shows	The Dentist
Guys	Diet soda
Money	Waking up
Videos	Homework
Sleeping	Tomato juice
More guys	Doing my hair
	Biting on a wood popsickle stick (nausea)

But while her social life improved over time, her problems with schoolwork continued. As expected, the school system was less intense than it had been in New Jersey. However, it became progressively more difficult for her. The educational social support system that had helped so much in Toronto and also in New Jersey was literally nonexistent here, but Stephanie had outgrown those needs. Still, her mother made it a habit of constantly monitoring the whole academic process. We met regularly with the teachers and staff to determine how to best juggle her curriculum. The challenge became greater each year. Her own ambitions, desires, and frustrations are revealed in her journal.

> *At 6D, I've got to go and finish my biology test.* [She was routinely given extra time to finish tests, often at home on an honor system.] *I'm going to fail, I know. There's definitely something wrong. I got two S's in English! What happened? I did something right for once. I got a 93 in Spanish. I think I did halfway decent in biology. I also did my English homework. I don't believe it, but I think I actually understood that crucible thing.*

Last night [her mother and I were away on a trip, and the person staying with them was unable to help Stephanie] *I studied from 7:00 to 11:30. I was dead. Then I tried to wake up at 5:30 to do more, but I couldn't. I ended up getting up at 6:30 instead, because the night before I studied from 5:00 until 10:00 and got up at 4:45. I think I'll go to bed early today. I'm going to fail geometry anyway. Miss Lott has been coming over to try to help me. Mr. Winthrop says I should drop out of geometry. I've got a 50 average. I am going to burn my report paper. Everybody else has 70's and 80's and even 90's. Oh, except a certain Marya. She's cool. I worked all day yesterday on a Napoleon report and missed my dental appointment. I think I failed all my quarterlies. Maya says if I get 75 on my Geometry, she'll take both of us out for pizza and a movie. But, if I get 80, she'll bring Dennis. I'm going to try and get an 80.*

I might go see Loverboy [the rock band]. *I hope I can go. Well they said no because it's a school night and my grades are too low. I'm upset now. I try hard. I dropped geometry, so now I can go riding every day like I'm supposed to. I think I passed the unit 22 test. Maybe even good like an 80 or 85-steak time! I wonder what Mom will do when I tell her about my 83. Mike says its good—only 2 points below Mark the brain. Ken says he got 62. I know the feeling.*

When we first moved back to Upstate New York, her mother discovered that there were no language classes for the early grades. To correct the situation, she and a friend organized Spanish classes. They solicited the help of a Spanish professor at a local college who assisted in interviewing and hiring a teacher. The school administration agreed to provide a classroom. They placed advertisements in the local newspaper, offering classes at ten dollars a semester. The response was more than sufficient. Stephanie and her sister both enrolled, and thus began their lifelong love of the language. So while her other grades sometimes suffered, Stephanie always did very well in Spanish.

Through it all, she attained a B average in grades seven and eight, slipping to a C in grades nine and ten. And each night, her mother was there helping her. Her literary skills continued their unabated development becoming, perhaps, just a little more descriptive and pointed. She wrote in her diary:

Marya won't tell me what she's gunna get me for Christmas. She did tell me it's blonde, but it's a rectangle and on T.V. I said hers was a rectangle, but it could be a circle. She asked if it was flat, and I told her it could be if you sat on it.

And later:

Mom made the grossest meatloaf—with ham! Yuck! I kept saying "Mighty dog." Geri made me shut up which is no easy task.

From her grade-nine journal:

Biology is really gross. The frogs smell rotton and their guts are all green and all sorts of lovely colors. I wanted to put one in Marya's locker but there's not much left of it. It's all skinned and one-half of it's inards are gone. On Thursday, Matt puked in the garbage can in biology—gross! Well, it's lunch time—bye.

My wife and I made a trip to Colorado for a few days, and Stephanie stayed with one family while her sister stayed with another. Stephanie's recollection goes like this:

I have to make chocolate cookies—by order. September 13—Those cookies look like warts! Maya threw one in my lunch. I hope I don't die. September 14-The cookies (warts) aren't bad.

The compromises and Stephanie's frustrations obviously required sacrifices, particularly for her sister. But we balanced things as best we could. We always sat near the front at movies, often well in front of the crowd.

Her sister never questioned why. We attempted to do things together that were active but attainable for Stephanie. We went bowling—which was difficult, but Stephanie managed—and roller skating, which she loved. She had learned to ice skate in Toronto, and whenever we could find an ice rink, we did that, too. A cross country ski area opened up nearby, and for a short time that became a family sport. And we took a chance and bought an outdoor badminton set. It was difficult, but to our surprise and pleasure, Stephanie was able to return the fly if it was hit high enough and straight in her direction.

Winter school breaks were spelled F-L-O-R-I-D-A. Both kids loved the water and the sun, but most of all Disney World and later, the Epcot Center. On one such trip, we visited Circus World, west of Orlando. At that time the park had the largest wooden structure roller coaster in the world. Stephanie had to try it. I was nominated by exception to go with her, and away we went. After the first dive, I felt like my eyes were up around my hairline. By the end of the ride, I was ecstatic to be alive. Somewhat unconsciously, I asked Stephanie if she wanted to go again. "Yes." Nineteen consecutive rides later, the answer finally came back, "No."

"Thank God," I said to myself, "I survived."

We worked to keep Christmas special. In her grade-nine journal, Stephanie wrote:

> *Christmas was OK. Mom wrapped a pair of pin PJ's in a tube made of cardboard and wrapped that in cloth. It looked like a huge fire cracker. I thought it was skis.*

I remember my father telling me when I got married what to expect of children. He related how when a child enters teenage years, the parents seem to become very dumb. A few years later, the parent somehow gains a tremendous amount of intelligence. This happened with Stephanie. As she entered adolescence, I somehow lost my intelligence. By the time she was fifteen, I had somewhat recovered. She wrote:

Dad returns from a three-week trip to China this Friday—good! I can't wait to see him—Like—I missed him this time.

We had never attended church with our children. About the time Stephanie turned sixteen, something told us we had made a serious error. In the continuing struggle she would face in life, we knew she would need a faith. After some discussion, we decided the time had come to attend church. We began to do so regularly. Little did we know then how critically important that step would be, not just for her, but for the whole family. As the burden of her cancer increased, she became more and more religious.

By the time she was fourteen, rock music had made its debut in our home and heavy metal was the variety of initial choice. Later, to our relief, her tastes mellowed, and I began taking her to rock concerts. The first one was a revelation to me. It was a group called Journey, accompanied by Bryan Adams. As we entered the stadium, I realized I was the oldest and baldest person among the fifty thousand there. I was careful to sit a few seats away from my passengers so as to not embarrass them!

Stephanie recalled the concert in her journal:

One thrilling thing we did last summer was to go to a concert, Journey and Bryan Adams (cute dude). Well, it was really loud. My Dad took Moi and four friends, but Dad liked it! It was so hot and our seats weren't. I was glad we had the binoculars! I missed Journey's entrance because I was in the "potty line." Good timing, Steph! Half of everybody yelled at me. Oh well. There were lots of decent guys around, so I was happy. (I was really glad we had the binoculars!) After all the music, it sounded like your head was under water. Then we went and blew more money on Burger King "Food."

I learned an important lesson at that concert. Several young people in their teens and early twenties came up to me and asked what I was doing there. At first, I misunderstood their question: Did they assume I did not trust my child, or that this was not my place? It all came clear when a girl of about eighteen approached me. I told her that I had brought my daughter and her friends. With tears in her eyes, she said, "You must really be a neat father." That kind of experience was repeated at subsequent concerts. For every one who asked, surely there were twenty who had the same thoughts without the inclination to express them. Kids are looking for love.

At subsequent assigned seat concerts, the usher guided us to the front row, even though our seats were toward the back. Upon attempting to point out the error, the usher said, "Well, from the looks of you, I thought you were a critic from the press."

Later we attended a great concert by the group Yes. Stephanie wrote:

I can't wait for the Yes concert. It will be cool. Our seats are in row O, if that means anything. Pretty bad, I think—binocular time. But we'll be closer than the Journey Concert.

From these concerts, I both developed more in common with Stephanie and also gained an appreciation of a different kind of music and came to better understand her point of view. She appreciated that and as a result, our relationship reached a new level. Some look in perplexity at the drug problem and the apparently unbridgeable gap between generations and wonder what to do about it. I doubt that the drug problem can be cured by cutting the South American or Asian supply lines. The cure will come when parents again accept responsibility for the family unit and do things with, rather than for, their children. Sharing music is a great place to start.

But first among all of Stephanie's activities was riding. Immediately following our move, she began riding at a nearby stable. Under excellent training, she blossomed. It was clearly time for her own horse. After searching for about two months, we found it. Capable of Belmont it was not, but it was what we needed. After searching her vocabulary for just the right name, the horse became Spinnaker, after the racing sail on a sailboat. The entry in her diary simply said, "My dream has come true."

We purchased riding gear and leather oil, and she kept that gear in top condition. And she quickly became an excellent rider. I was shocked when the instructor said, "Well, it's time for her to start jumping." I could not conceive of how she would be able to follow a course, let alone line up for the jumps. The answer came from the instructor. He would position Stephanie and her horse several yards away from the fence. Since Stephanie had trouble figuring out how to position herself, another person would stand on the opposite side of the fence. Stephanie would then aim her horse for the person. That strategy worked. Within weeks, she was taking jumps regularly. Later, she was able to follow a very complicated course. How she did this remains a mystery, but she never erred. I would often stand by her as she struggled to follow the course of the other riders with her eye. However, once in the ring, her confidence would swell.

The ribbons quickly began to accumulate. After a time, we strung two wires in a V in her room. By the time she was sixteen, there were forty-one ribbons on these wires. At fifteen, she attended a major show at Cornell University. She came home with a fistful of ribbons. She wrote in her diary:

Today Gary [her coach] *said I really did good, especially over jumps. He wants me to get a show horse. I said I wanted to keep Spin. He even used me as an example—fun.*

And a few weeks later:

At Sunday's show, I got 2–1st, 1–3rd and 2––4th, 1–6th and a championship. They gave me a little pewter plate for that. Gary says I've got to sell Spinny. I hope somebody will take good care of her.

Separately, we had also been approached by the stable. It was time for an upgrade, as Stephanie was becoming professional. She needed a faster sail. *This summer,* I thought.

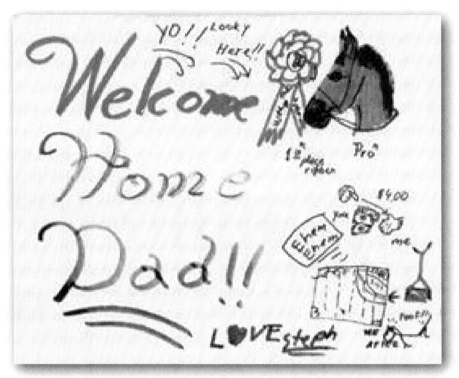

More ribbons – faster sail than Spinnaker required

But riding was only part of the scene. The stable had a very active summer camp offering riding, swimming, and simply good fun. Stephanie attended this camp each summer, and it was here that she had her only close call—which made us think again about our original decision to come down on the side of risk. Her notes tell the story best:

On Sunday, Heather and I were doing the hunt course. It was cool until Spinny ran me into a tree. Was I in pain! I didn't want to take the corner so sharp and ended up going straight. My arms are all scratched up and my lip went through my bottom braces. Then I had to pull a thorn out of my shoulder and go to the emergency room and get one out of my head—t h r i l l s!

In April 1984, Stephanie wrote:

I messed up my knee. I pulled my riding boot off by way of the edge of the step. I'm limping around now and feeling severe pain in it. Mom's taking me to see the doctor today. I hope I get crutches.

In late May she wrote:

Dr. McAfree says it's OK to wear the bandage. It's weird because I'll be walking along and it will bend the wrong way and I'll yell.

Too much riding, it appeared, was taking its toll on those young knee joints. On the doctor's advice, she had to temporarily give up riding, much to her disappointment. In spite of the pain, Stephanie insisted on playing in the marching band parade. This was a spring event our town had hosted for years. Each year, it seemed to grow in size and notoriety. High school marching bands from all over the state would attend. So Stephanie applied her knee support and, in visible pain, marched her way down State Street, proudly playing her flute in the school marching band.

For Memorial Day weekend we met the Tighlmans, our prior New Jersey neighbors, in New Hampshire. They had moved to Boston, and our families met at a beautiful old summer home of their family. It was like old times with everybody, parents and children, playing and talking with one another.

We had fun with the Tighlmans. I slept thirteen hours on Sunday. Dad says I looked well rested.

CHAPTER 6

Cancer

● ● ●

Dad's going to Harvard for six weeks. Those Dad steelers! I wish he'd cut that out. I wonder if they'll raid the dorms and have fire alarms.

IN THE SPRING OF 1984, I had enrolled in the Harvard Advanced Management Program in anticipation of greater responsibilities at work. I had been fortunate in my career selection. After graduating from college, my first job was in the producing oilfields of Western Canada. As the job developed, I found myself more and more in the northern parts of Alberta and British Columbia. Not a lot of time passed before I realized that God or whoever else was responsible had placed newly discovered oil in the more remote locations. I recall one night in midwinter driving my company pickup truck along the frozen Athabasca River on my way to the nearest town, some fifty miles away. In the winter, the river was the only passable road. About halfway through the journey, my vehicle began to stall. The temperature outside was a cool -60°F. For reasons unknown to me, the truck kept on. If it had stalled, Stephanie would not have been born and this book would not have been written. During that trip I decided that I was best suited to another environment.

A few months later I accepted a position as application engineer with an industrial machinery manufacturer in Toronto. Shortly thereafter, I knew I had found my niche. Eighteen years later, I was to attend Harvard as part of a program to prepare me as a contender for the presidency of the fine company that employed me.

The Sunday I left, we went to church and lunch. Stephanie recorded the event in a note to a friend:

Church was terrible today! We had to eat bread and drink grape juice! It dried my oral cavity out. Then we went to a classy restaurant for a buffet. The guy who cut the roast beef was pretty cute.

I was thrilled about the refreshing interlude at Harvard, broken into two segments—one in 1984 and a second one a year later. After having been away from college for over twenty years, a short return to the academic environment and particularly Harvard was inviting.

But even before I left, we had become worried. In spite of prescribed exercises, Stephanie's knee was not improving. Five days after I started classes, we had her leg x-rayed. The doctor spotted a calcium deposit the size of a quarter next to her knee. Her mother explained Stephanie's earlier retinoblastoma, and his response was that these occurrences would not be connected since it had been too many years since her first cancer. We discussed his conclusions, and my wife then called Dr. Ellsworth. He asked only one question: "Which side is it on?" With her response that it was on the same side as her regular eye, he urged her to have a CAT scan done as soon as possible.

Her mother arranged for a CAT scan as quickly as could be scheduled, which was the following week. I made tentative arrangements to leave Harvard.

On the day of the CAT scan, I waited by the phone in my dorm for what seemed to be an eternity. Finally, late in the afternoon, with terrible anxiety, I called the doctor. The call was forwarded to him in the x-ray room. His voice was low. Stephanie was in the next room. The printout was just coming off the computer.

"Yes," he said, "there are lesions, at least one and perhaps more." My wife came to the phone, and I told her I was coming home. Knowing how much I was enjoying Harvard and that I had been there only ten days, she suggested I stay on. But I could never have done that. The doctor and I then spoke again. He suggested that we take Stephanie to Roswell Park Hospital in Buffalo. "No," I responded. Our experience and decision years earlier had left a clear impression. We would either go for the best treatment we knew—and go for it fast—or we would do nothing at all.

I was packed and leaving the parking lot at Harvard within a half-hour. I can barely recall the trip home, except for two incidents. A State Police trooper stopped me for speeding. Not waiting for him to approach my car, I went directly to his.

"My daughter has cancer, and I'm going home," I said.

"She isn't going to die tonight, is she?" he asked.

I walked back to my car and drove off without even answering. Later, I stopped and called home. My wife relayed the story about the day. Stephanie had her friend Suzy accompany her for the CAT scan. Upon receiving the results, her mother told her that while we could not be sure, there was at least a tumor and that it could be cancer. They then concluded that if it was cancer, we would go to New York as before and have it taken care of.

Only later, when her mother told her I was leaving Harvard and coming home, did Stephanie begin to cry. Then she went to her room to study for a final exam the next day—an exam she would not take.

Much later, Stephanie told her mother that in the early days of her knee problem she'd had a dream that she once again had cancer.

When Stephanie was young, we had debated many times as to whether to tell her she had had cancer. I was insistent we not tell her, since I felt that she had enough burdens in her life. Her mother felt that this was her life and her body and that she had a right to know. My position prevailed. When Stephanie was thirteen, however, she drew her mother into a discussion about cancer. Stephanie said what a difficult thing it would be to have cancer. Her mother decided the time had come and told Stephanie she had already had the disease. Later, Stephanie told a close friend she was very disturbed that we had not told her before. "Didn't they think I could have handled it?" she asked. "It was my body." In retrospect, I was indeed wrong. It was her body, and she did have a right to know. I decided not to make that mistake again.

I arrived home at midnight, and we made reservations on a flight to New York the next morning. We had no appointment and did not even have the name of a doctor. All we knew was that we were going to Sloan Kettering Memorial Institute. I vowed that night on the long drive home from Boston that we would not make the error we had made over sixteen years earlier. We had already lost too much time.

It may seem odd to not consider medical costs, as Sloan Kettering was and is a highly rated cancer clinic and obviously could be very expensive. However, the company that employed me had a special medical plan for vice presidents and officers. In addition to normal coverage, we had an additional plan that covered all medical costs, regardless of amount. So the only costs to be absorbed personally were travel and related expenses.

I also called the man we would once more come to rely on, Dr. Ellsworth. I said we would be at his office in a few hours and asked that he have a reference for us at Sloan Kettering, next to the Eye Institute at Columbia Presbyterian Hospital, where he now maintained his practice.

As we were preparing to leave for the airport, Stephanie's friends came by to walk with her to school. "I can't take the exam," she said. "I have to go to New York because I have a tumor, but I'll be back in three days." My heart would not let me correct her.

The word *cancer* stimulates the darkest, most negative feelings in people. The obvious initial reactions are fear and confusion. Nothing I or anyone can say or reduce to print will change that. The best course of action, we found, was to get the best information possible from friends, associates, and doctors, confirm it if possible, and then act on it. Inaction only multiplies the fear. Action, in and of itself, reduces the confusion and fear. At least something is being done.

By 2:30 p.m., we had met Stephanie's doctor at Sloan Kettering, Dr. Caparros-Sissons, and had the diagnosis—osteogenic sarcoma of the tibia, the bone just below the knee: Stephanie had bone cancer. We were referred to Dr. Ralph Marcove for reasons we found confusing at that moment but which became clear somewhat later. After an inspection he said, "I can save that leg." *If we could get Stephanie into the hospital*, he'd said, he would arrange for a biopsy four days later.

Things were happening too fast. We felt swept along by the flow of events. With Dr. Caparros-Sissons we had openly discussed the chemotherapy treatment involved. Stephanie wanted to know her chances of surviving. The doctor openly told her "between 50 and 80 percent." In those terribly emotional moments, Stephanie must have missed the point that to control bone cancer, the affected area must be removed—amputated. Of Dr. Marcove's comments, she later wrote:

> *At first, I thought the chemo would kill the tumor, then I would go home. That was why I was taking it. When Dr. Marcove said, we're going to save that leg, I didn't quite get it. Brilliant to not tell me.*

Hearing Dr. Marcove say the words, "If we can get her in the hospital" raised a red flag for me. The next morning, I went to hospital admittance and literally created an emergency, using doctors' names as references, and returning to the clerk every five minutes until I got a bed for Stephanie. I found out later that I had done in a few hours what can take three to five days at Sloan or many other hospitals.

If we had not pushed as we had, Stephanie probably would have had her biopsy ten days later. It was not the fault of the doctors. They did not run the hospital. I also cannot say that ten days would or would not have made any difference. What I do know is that the osteogenic sarcoma did not return. We also had the satisfaction of doing something.

In between our visits to Drs. Sissons and Marcove, we had been able to find a private area on an outdoor patio in the children's hospital section. Stephanie cried, and her mother held her as only a mother can. She wanted to know if she would die. "I don't know, but we will find out after the biopsy," her mother said.

Many people make the assumption—as I had years earlier—that it is better for the patient to not know the truth. This may be OK in some cases, but on balance, I disagree. In Stephanie's case, it would have been disastrous. In the last phases of her illness she had to deal with a doctor who was not being truthful and any semblance of credibility was shattered. Stephanie had no use for him and he knew it. With Stephanie, you knew where you stood and she expected the same. By being completely truthful with Stephanie on the first day, we established a level of trust and credibility that grew and paid dividends until our child took her last breath.

That night we went out to dinner and bought Stephanie a huge lobster dinner. She loved lobster and ate it all. We then went to our new home, the Ronald McDonald House, at 419 East Eighty-Sixth Street, and the relative security of being with those who knew what we knew.

A few hours before her biopsy, Stephanie wrote to her friends Marya and Karen:

Hello, you Upstate dwellers. I'm in room 512B at Memorial Hospital. They give you a cute little TV. It's hard to see Jamison Parker on a 3x5" screen. My stupid knee's giving me an immense amount of pain. Those ultrageeks won't give me any codeine, cause I have surgery in two hours. They wouldn't give me pain killer, so I've been soaking in my tub for the last half hour. Mom spent last night here in an extra cot. Dad's back at the Ronald McDonald House. It's really nice there. Atari and a cool stereo. There's this guy here who I call "the Prep." He walks like Betty Crocker too. He's so airheaded! He needs to learn a few terms. He's pretty OK though. Deep brown eyes—dark hair and a pink oxford shirt. It's so gross (not the food) they make you excreaterize in this florescent blue-green plastic thing! They've got to weigh it—even the poo-poo. It stinks up the bathroom and makes fish feel like puking.

Oh, they're gunna put an IV tube in me!! Get me out of here! Rescue me G.B. [Karen]. Poor little Fish.

Well, I don't know exactly how long I'll be here—maybe even a week more. It takes them forever to figure out what's wrong with the bone they take out. I would like you to know I do miss you very much. Fish (even the kissing ones in the playroom) have feelings! Say happy birthday to Egroeg [George, a friend, spelled backward]. *I'm sorry 'cause I thought I only stay for three days.*

Well, there's not much else to report at this time. Good luck on your Algebra Regents! I'm sure you'll pass. Love, Steph the Fish

Stephanie's biopsy operation was late in the day. While she was still in recovery, Dr. Marcove came with the news. He was positive it was malignant. The biopsy would prescribe the type of chemotherapy. He was not optimistic about the long-term prospects. He suspected the cancer would recur, probably in the lungs. He urged us to push Dr. Sissons to start chemotherapy as soon as possible. We told Stephanie what we knew as soon as the effects of her anesthesia had sufficiently subsided. She was calm, her internal toughness ready for the fight.

The biopsy was far more painful than we had anticipated. As she was recovering from the anesthetic, Stephanie at first refused medication. By the time she agreed to accept relief, she was in excruciating pain. The prescribed drug was morphine, which is effective only when pain is entering the threshold level. Since it was now far beyond that, she was given a large dose and, even then, significant time went by before she was calm. This was our first experience in observing her strength in handling pain.

Stephanie had an old Walkman that she had brought with her. I had bought her some funny posters about rock and roll, some notepads, and a tape for her to listen to. I called her friend Marya and asked her to get some friends together that day and record a tape for Stephanie. They did that night and we had it sent by Federal Express. The subject of the tape, made by about eight friends, was "Where is Stephanie?" They looked in her fish tank, toilet bowl, down the Jenn Air stove, in the fireplace, the oven, the cupboards, the fridge, the toaster, the microwave, and so on. They also decided that since she could not come to her animals, they would bring them to her. On the tape is the bird chirping, the dog barking, and the fish tank bubbling. It was hilarious and gave Stephanie a great lift. These are the things, I found, which make all the difference—doing the unexpected at the right time.

Before her operation, she asked if I would get her a new Walkman if her tumor was malignant (a biopsy is necessary to be certain of malignancy). I said yes. The day after her operation, even before we had the official report back, I bought her the best I could find. I will never forget the beautiful hug and kiss she gave me when I brought it into her room. She was still in pain and immobile, but she raised herself off that bed and threw her arms around me and kissed me.

As soon as friends and acquaintances began to hear about Stephanie's condition, the cards and gifts began to pour in. Her room at Sloan and later at home became literally full of stuffed toys. One, a big fat cat that I bought for her was one of her real favorites. She called it Sylvia and I called it Templeton after the fat rat in the movie *Charlotte's Web*. Whenever the pain became extreme, she would hug that cat. She rarely cried.

One of the frustrations felt at times by friends, particularly those far away, is a feeling of helplessness. So they sent encouragement and love. This whole process of support was tremendously therapeutic for all of us.

Stephanie was on the mend within a few days, and her treatment protocol had been established. We were becoming more familiar with the ordeal of dealing with this disease. We were moving "inside." Having been a nurse, my wife was able to sort out what at times appeared to me to be terrible confusion. The treatment was to be some heavy chemotherapy for eight weeks on an outpatient basis, followed by an extensive leg operation, followed by more chemotherapy. The second treatment period would last either four or nine months, depending on the tumor's reaction to the initial chemo. Mixed within this would be a baffling number of tests, x-rays, and other kinds of treatment. We did not know then just how uncertain it would become.

A vision of the inner Stephanie began to come through—that loving, positive, courageous sixteen-year-old who was already honing the ability to simply turn off, shut out, or forget anything that was no longer possible. She was not one to bemoan her fate. In the first of her multiple body scans, where she had to be in the room alone, she poked her head out and said to her mother, "Hey, Mom, this is going to be forty-five minutes—may as well go and enjoy yourself."

Just before her chemotherapy was to begin, she wrote to Maya:

Thanks a lot for the group tape, card and letter. I feel much better. I resent being sucked down the Jenn Air fan. Not humorous! I hate to say, but you probably already know you can look down the Jenn-Air all you want—but the vent goes to New York City the whole summer. Todo el verano! Lorac Noznag [Maya's mother's name spelled backward] *says you can visit. Do if at all possible—PLEASE! And take me home.*

I'm soooooooooo—sorry to miss your grad bash. We've still got your b'day + grad peace offerings at home in some remote area. Well, Happy Graduation!!! Can you handle a party without me? I'm not so important.

So John has taken an interest in me has he? He's mine. I saw him first. He doesn't ski! Tell him I'm in NYC getting treatment for cancer and could write to him. Watch you guys get married! I'll tell him about you and Pete and Tim and Danny. You heartbreaker, man stealer. I'd better stop before I get unintentionally and verbally cruel.

I'm an outpatient now and am sitting on a bed in Ronald McDonald House. Mom's in La Cocina cooking dinner. I've got my cancer leg on two pillows and am listening to Led Zepplin Vol. II in my Toshiba walk thing. Do you like Zep? I used to hate them. I still hate their noisy ones, none of which are on this fine tape (Thank God!) I'm sick of all of mine. Do you ever get that feeling? WAPP 103.5 is a lot like WCMF. You can't get 95.7? Try WOUR in Cortland or some place. I could hear it by your place.

The crud I go through (NYC as I view it) Tests—sharable with others of the same species. Biopsy—consists of stitches, swelling, pain, non-walkability, absence of a piece of bone and all feeling (outer epidermis) of left knee (the surgery). Also, buns hurt from sitting and lying around. Bone Scan—injection of radioactive liquid kept in a metal box (impressive). After two hours and as many cups of H2O, laying on hard table for prolonged period of time (1 hour) holding still, as scanner slowly scans the whole skeletal formation for other tumors. Painless, yet rather meaningless + DULL!

Gut Scan—injection of same description as above. Two days + many glasses of H2O, laying on a table (hard) as scanner takes 1-1/2 hours. To scan most of innards for tumors. Again, painless, meaningless + DULL (as never before!) Lung Test—breathe into silly gray tasteless mouthpiece. Kill your lungs + get a clip on your nose and feel really foolish. Also change your mouth size 8 sizes larger.

Well, that's all that's new. I hope you feel better than I (not really bad). Write back. Ronald McDonald House 419 E. 86 St. New York, NY 10028 No more hospital! Lov Choco Chip Cookie Caper Steph

We were trying to decide how we could best handle the family situation. We concluded that my wife would be with Stephanie constantly. I would do my best to take care of my other daughter and keep working. We would find someone to help with our home life. If possible, I would come to New York and my wife would come home on weekends.

It soon became obvious that exchanging locations for the weekend was highly impractical. So she would stay in New York for two weeks during chemotherapy, and they would then be home for one. And on it went.

The weeks and months ahead would see us dealing with things on a day-to-day basis as we learned that the chemotherapy schedule placed neatly on a piece of paper bears little relationship to reality. Scheduling, low blood counts, and the like make the treatment process uncertain at best. But as we settled into a routine of dealing with rapidly changing events, Stephanie gained in strength and courage. The more people commented on her courage and her open approach to cancer, the more she gained self-confidence and an increasing commitment to continue, and the circle of confidence and reinforcement grew, expanded, and strengthened.

CHAPTER 7

More Trials, More Victories

● ● ●

THE ROLLER-COASTER RIDE CONTINUED AS the chemo went on. And we began to see firsthand the severe side effects of chemotherapy. We needed to affirm our earlier decision to take the aggressive route. Stephanie later wrote in her diary about the chemo:

> *Staying up to the microscopic hours of the morning is no problem because of all the methotrexate I've received. Getting up every four hours to take three or more sodiumbicarbonates. If beer doesn't make you burp, these WILL! This doesn't compliment the fact that you've been drinking 3000 cc's to get the crap out of your system and are nauseated.*
>
> *Methotrexate is bright, vibrant fluorescent yellow, and takes four hours to run. You get to watch the wretched stuff go down the tube till it hits you, wait a few minutes and then start to heave. This is by far the easiest chemo I have been put through. No side effects such as hair loss (major league shed syndrome), severe loss of appetite, or intestinal coma.*
>
> *BCD causes these wonderful benefits. It caused my intestines to go on strike once. Or was that cysplatinum? This wonder drug runs for seven hours. You get to the hospital before anyone's turned on the lights. You leave at 6:30 p.m. They give you a whole bunch of other things with it. A few days later you wish you were dead. Hell sounds fine compared to this. I was afraid I'd kill myself. I found myself up in the attic looking for Dad's hunting guns. If I found one, I don't know that I'd be here at the present.*

On BCD, I remember the wonderful benefits. I couldn't force my-self to eat. The nutrition department was threatening me with TPN. That's when you're the lucky recipient of yet another tube. This one goes down your nose to your stomach. I weighed about 75 pounds according to Mom. I got home and couldn't look at myself in the mirror. I wore size one clothes as compared to sixe three, and could have been from Ethiopia.

Food was repulsive to me, like an ugly design on a plate. You wouldn't eat the pattern on a plate, why eat the food? I'd swallow a crust, and back up it would arrive in a matter of seconds.

Mom says I was asking if I'd die. I don't remember that.

As the reaction to the chemo intensified, we pondered what to do. With some hesitancy, we made contact with several treatment centers in Southern California. These centers provide a natural treatment system, concentrating on vitamins, ground-up fruit pits, and similar edible earth-born items. However, this kind of holistic medicine is generally not endorsed by the US medical profession. These centers also seemed to have few statistics on survival rate. They suggested, however, that we come out for an evaluation.

My sister called to see how we were doing. I told her of our dilemma, and she related a story of a friend who had bone cancer, was declared terminal, and proceeded to Mexico for this type of treatment. This had been several years earlier, and he had apparently beaten the disease and was in good health. I also was following the progress of an older cousin. Several years earlier, he had contracted prostate cancer. Chemotherapy had been successful, but the cancer had recently returned. He had a full physical at a nearby cancer center, and they had advised that he not attempt treatment. The cancer, this time in the bone, had progressed too far in their estimation. He and his wife flew to San Diego, proceeded to Tijuana, and he started treatments. He had been given six months to live, and it was now one year later. The cancer was disappearing. He continued to live for at least a decade, perhaps longer.

We were deeply torn. Stephanie's treatments were much worse than we had imagined. The doctors advised that Stephanie's reactions were not abnormal. They had also made it clear early on that strict adherence to treatment protocol was a prerequisite to our chances for success. There was literally no time to travel to California to evaluate our options without stopping treatments in New York. We had heard of successes from the natural treatment regimen. But the successes we were aware of had been all with older people, where cancer tends to progress much more slowly. But still, they were successes.

After some heavy discussions, we decided that the risk of stepping outside the established medical system was one we were not prepared to take. We went on. Whether we were right or wrong, we will never know. I do not regret our decision. If we had taken the unconventional route and it had failed, I do not know that I could have lived with that burden.

Stephanie's demeanor remained bright. Having lost her hair, she happily collected a variety of wigs. Between treatments, she and her friends attended a local street dance. Stephanie, on crutches, in a blonde wig with a fancy bandanna around it, stayed up until the wee hours of the morning. Later, back in New York, she wrote to Marya:

Marya: Hello. I got your letter a couple days ago, but I felt like poo-poo. I am now returning your endeavor. I'm glad you were thrilled to see me. I was as much (or more) to see you, but don't get emotionally aroused during a long-awaited greeting.

I almost passed out this morning. It was too hot in the bathroom, and I got out of the tub too fast. It was weird—everything was black. I'm fine now.

I won't be back to stay until November! I'm not coming home this weekend 'cause I'm coming home for two weeks next Wednesday. So you can throw a bash for me.

I've received a lot of peace offerings from my Dad's friends—a huge bowl of fruit and flowers. We let people have some 'cause we could never finish it ourselves. I also got two tapes from my cousin.

Mom wants me to go shopping for a wig, but I don't feel good enough to; how embarrassing. I'll probably be sorry when I'm totally bald. If I'm home, don't call me baldy—OK?

On Monday and Tuesday I get eight hours of IV fluid! Eight hours each day! It gives you nausea too! Boy, will I be cheerful when I get home.

Write back or die. Love Steph

A few weeks later, she wrote to her Spanish teacher:

Dear Mrs. Wilson: Hi, it's me. You said you had some interest in what was to become of me, so I am writing to inform your thoughtful self. I'm all right except for my knee. In case you haven't heard, I've got bone cancer. I'm undergoing chemotherapy until November. I probably won't be attending school much, so to accommodate, I'm staying back one year.

Oh, this cancer stuff. They're gunna put a piece of scrap metal (fake knee joint) in the week after next. I'll be unable to run until I'm re-born. Gross! No more gym class maybe. Sorry I can't compose this literature En Espanol!

Well, they torture one with lots of IV's and stuff. For example, high dose methotrexate is the yellow stuff that kills cancer cells and Vincristine is one that helps. So what they do is IV methotrexate into you for four hours—dull! Then I've gotta get that out of my system, so I drink three quarts of water every day for three days—tough. Then the day after the IV I get an injection of Vincristine which has various side effects such as numbness, pain in every single joint in your entire body, mouth sores and—yes, hair loss. I'm a blonde now—$15, K-Mart special. Don't say much if anybody asks—I mean the wig. As far as you know, I dyed it— OK? If this stuff wasn't so side effect, I'd be all right (along with about 2000 others!) Some they can't save. I know a 4-year-old who's gunna die—bummer! I really hope you don't move. I won't let you. Do write back if you wish (please do). Love Steph

The time for leg surgery had arrived. Rather than amputate, they would take out a section of bone on each side of the knee, then remove the knee itself and replace the whole section with a titanium knee joint with spikes extending into the tibia and femur. This process (which was breakthrough at the time), pioneered by Dr. Marcove, would save her leg and a good amount of our daughter's dignity. It was a terribly complex ten-hour operation. Stephanie went in with calmness and great confidence. Her courage, good humor, and openness were becoming well-known in the children's pediatric section of Sloan Kettering. The night before the operation, her mother asked if she wanted her to stay, and Stephanie declined. She was fine.

The ten-hour operation became an all-day ordeal, as we first waited four hours for her to go to the operating room, and then too many hours thereafter. Complications had occurred: her femur had cracked in the replacement process. Stephanie now had a broken leg that would have to heal.

She had been tipped off by a nurse before surgery to ask for water as soon as she awoke from surgery. This, she was told, would get her out of the recovery room and back to her regular room more quickly. She was back before the room nurses were ready for her. One nurse in the recovery room said, "I've never seen anyone recover so quickly. She was barely awake when she asked for water."

Her recovery was rapid at first—but then it began to drag on as the incision refused to heal. Bending her leg was very painful, but she never asked for medication. She just wanted it to heal so she could ride her horse again. Later, she wrote of that experience in her diary:

Another measurably painful experience was when Dr. Marcove would come in the room and have to bend the leg to stop adhesions from forming. I'm sure they could hear me screaming down the hall a piece. He'd pick up the whole leg and hold it above the joint and let it fall. I could feel as well as hear the adhesions breaking. It sounded like popcorn. It felt painful beyond belief. He said it broke his heart to do that.

But as time dragged on, she wrote Marya:

I think I'm gunna be stuck in here forever. Now I might get plastic sur-gery on my leg. I give up!

And she kept her sense of humor. Later, she wrote:

In that six weeks, I had an IV in my arm every day except one. That day I raced down the halls with my new found freedom—a self-propelled wheelchair. Mobility on my own. This must be what it's like to drive a car, I thought.

Two weeks following the operation, her sister and I went to New York for the weekend. What started out to be as much a family a weekend as possible under the circumstances became very difficult. On Sunday morning, we received word that my company president had died suddenly, following emergency surgery. Her sister and I had to return home immediately in the presence of more sadness. We had lost a true personal and family friend, one of the most caring people I have ever known. Stephanie cried deeply; she really liked this man.

During her healing, she kept watch on the doctors and wrote:

There was this Russian guy, Dr. No. We thought he was a spy or some-thing. One time Dr. No came into the room looking for the other doctors and almost looked under the bed. Problem, Dr. No? I only thought this— they're not hiding under the bed.

Finally, six weeks after her operation, Stephanie had healed enough to come home. While I picked them up at the airport, some good friends put a bunch of "Welcome Home, Stephanie" banners, balloons, and streamers across the front of our home. When she saw it, she allowed her one-sided, sly grin and said, "What's all this hoopla for?" Once inside, everybody hugged everybody. Our phone rang constantly, and visitors dropped in for the next two weeks while she was home. Her core of deep friends, adults and teenagers, was developing.

Shortly after her operation, when she was still in the hospital, we were given tough news. A postoperative analysis had shown that the sarcoma had not responded well to the initial chemotherapy. Rather than having the relative luxury of being treated to a lighter form of chemo for a short period, Stephanie would have to receive very difficult treatments until July of the following year. We were to be faced with a continuation of chemo products with names like Cysplatinum, BCD, and Vincristine.

She took the news in a matter-of-fact way; it was something she could not change, so she would not be bothered further by it.

The process of returning to normal meant relearning to walk. Unable to negotiate the stairs, she was at first confined to her room, where she kept herself busy. She wrote to her friends, listened to her stereo, and played with her birds and fed her fish. Invariably, as I drove in the driveway after work, she would be waving both hands at me from her window. She persevered, however, and in a few weeks was becoming ambulatory again. As Stephanie began to use her leg, we discovered it was about one and a half inches too short, and not straight—that is, her foot "toed in" about fifteen degrees, causing her to trip on her other foot if she was not careful.

At a later time, she asked, "Could this all be corrected with a second operation?" "Yes," was the doctor's response. "Fine," she said in turn. The decision was as simple as that. In the meantime, we had all of her left shoes raised. But it was better than an amputation.

Still, her activities were severely limited. She would never be able to run or ride her bike again. Swimming would be a problem, although she was able to continue to a degree. And horseback riding was absolutely out on strict orders by her doctor. But more on that later.

Once more, Stephanie adapted. Thanks to some good friends at my workplace and elsewhere, she began to receive letters and cards from a lot of people from all over the world. Through various sources, she found pen pals in England, Ireland, Sweden, and many parts of the United States.

She also became much more interested in music, and her interests changed to a mellower, deeper type of music where each word carried special meaning. She began to like Kate Bush, a beautiful English singer, and became attracted to the music of the famous group U2. Through her, we as a family also developed a better appreciation of this music.

Obviously, with all of the chemotherapy ahead of her, it was impractical for her to take her junior year in 1984–1985. This was the year to attempt to stabilize her condition. High school and college could be resumed later, we said.

So we went into the coming months with the prospect of a lot of turmoil and braced ourselves for it. There were many times when, due to chemotherapy, my travel requirements, unexpected sickness, or simply the need to get away for an hour, we urgently needed the help of friends. We found, not to our surprise, that there are "friends" and there are deep friends. "Friends," we found, are people who you call for urgent help, and they say that if it weren't for their hair appointment, they'd be happy to help; but how about tomorrow, because they're free then. A deep friend says, "I have nothing planned, and I'll be over in fifteen minutes," and then proceeds to cancel the hair appointment and never mentions that there was one in the first place. We had several deep friends, thank God.

I have given a lot of thought to this difference and have concluded that people who come up short do so not out of lack of desire, but because their maturity is not developed well enough to understand when a friend really needs help. As a result, they put themselves before their friend. A deep friend has developed this maturing, and unless he or she is simply being taken advantage of, will respond every time. And deep friends will do so not thinking that they are doing a big favor; helping is simply the right priority for them.

One of our most loyal deep friends had two young children, and she never failed us. I recall one morning our other daughter was not feeling well and was unable to go to school. I called the friend with two young children and asked if she could help. She responded that she had nothing planned and would be over in a few minutes. I later found out that she had another engagement, which she canceled to help us.

Even though she was unable to attend school, Stephanie wanted to be able to enter her junior year the following September. So she again took the two subjects for which she had not written exams and the following spring easily passed both.

And she rode her horse!

Whenever she had the strength, and sometimes when she didn't, she rode. The operation had resulted in some loss of feeling and control in her foot, but she accommodated. We took her regularly, sometimes so she could be with the horse but usually to ride. Since jumping takes knee control, she was no longer able to do that but did everything else. And she looked as she always had in the saddle. So Dr. Marcove, if you are reading this, you know that we totally disobeyed your orders. But, somehow, I think you will agree that we did the right thing.

CHAPTER 8

Seizing the Moment

• • •

WHEN COMMODITIES OR RESOURCES ARE assumed to be in plentiful supply, society places a lower value on them. So it seems also with life. When one assumes that it will go on, seemingly forever, each day does not carry the value it does when its duration becomes questionable. We found with ourselves and with Stephanie a much more intense appreciation of life. Stephanie had little patience for trivia or people who dwelled on it. The same was true for movies. She watched only those with character and substance. Because of their subtleties, she came to love Peter Sellers's movies and Monty Python shows. Her personal relationships took the same route. As a result, each period became more important and later, more precious. She wrote in her diary:

> *Poor Mrs. Becker, yes, my beloved Keyboarding instructor has the elite privilege of listening to me complain. Know what? She said she doesn't mind! Sometimes, she even agrees with me. It's easier to communicate with humans of the adult variety. They're not so immature.*
>
> *On the Oprah show, they interviewed ladies that turned to prostitution to feed their families. They asked if they thought this profession was acceptable. Why don't they ask the clients if they think they themselves are being acceptable, or get some guy up there?*

Christmas is special for most families. Starting in 1984, it became special and important—and by 1986, it became precious. Each year we performed the ritual of cutting our own Christmas tree, and 1984 was no exception.

Characteristically, we would decide on tree height and needle length a few days before the outing. By the fateful day, we all had fairly hardened positions on each. We would troupe into the grove, each pick and stand by an entirely different kind of tree of every description, and then we would negotiate with one another until one by one, each gave in to one.

Tempers would ebb and flow, and in the last instance, everyone would suddenly feel good about having picked just the right tree. It was tough for Stephanie in 1984 because she had lost muscle control and feeling in her ankle, which would often turn over on its side. She also had a full-length removable cast on her leg. Nonetheless, the importance of getting just the right tree overcame the problem, and she was out there with us as always. We went a shorter distance into the grove because of her condition but went through the same negotiating process. When we came in with our tree, the grove owner casually asked Stephanie what was wrong with her leg. Stephanie, equally casually, responded, "I have bone cancer."

The owner was speechless. When we were all in the car, Stephanie asked, "What was wrong with him?"

We made the most of Christmas despite Stephanie's returning to New York before the New Year to resume treatment. But at least we had Christmas together. The weeks to come would be defined by a continuation of shuttling to New York and dealing with the unknown. Note writing became the norm:

2/15/85
Dad,

Somebody has to clean the fish tank and get credit for the music box before the 18th. And Sunday would be an easier day to leave at 6:00 a.m., so I can get to see Spinny. OK? Me P.S. Tom T. Hall is a very bad influence on your already pretty bad musical interests! He also needs smiling lessons.

In a subsequent set of chemotherapy, she had a reaction that caused her eye to rotate in until her pupil was inside her eyelid, and she could not see. Fearing permanent blindness, she said to her mother, "I can't go on."

An emergency injection of a counteracting drug reversed the process, and in a few hours, her eye was properly positioned again. And she went on. To occupy her time, she turned to crafts and made gifts for her friends. For me, she made a stuffed alligator, calling it Prepus Maximus.

And we increased our bird population. One of the managers at the McDonald House kept doves in the cage. Copulation, cage style, produced two eggs, and as a result, the birds had to be separated. He offered one to Stephanie, and we didn't have the heart to say no. Stephanie wrote, "I asked him how much for it and he said a kiss—paid for."

In New York, I rented a car and drove home with Derrick, the dove, which cooed continuously. I stopped at the famous Roscoe Diner and shut the car off on that cold winter night, hoping that when I came back out, the frigid weather would have shrunk its larynx. No such luck.

Through the kindness of the doctors, we were able to bend some rules, and we arranged to go to Hawaii during school break. Weak, very thin, and pale, Stephanie still handled the long trip. Because of the chemo, she was able to go in the sun only for very short periods. Chemotherapy has the effect of weakening those chemicals in the blood that protect against sunburn. But we made the most of it in a beautiful condo on Kaanapali Bay, Maui. Stephanie kept her humor. She wrote Marya from LAX:

It's now 4:30 p.m. where you are, and 1:30 here. We'll be there in five hours. On the other plane, they served food, kinda real lasting too. We're gonna suffer through dinner too. It's an air food day, I guess. How to fly though a meal. The day just flew by.

And from Maui:

Like this condo is fantastic. It's got two bedrooms and two potty rooms, kitchen, breakfast nook, living room and a TV. Oh, there's this thing in the potty rooms. It's called a bidet. It's a permanent you know what cleaner—gross!! It looks like a toilet with a fountain in it.

Stephanie loved Maui. We walked the beaches as much as we could and drove around the island. Our condo faced west, and each night we had a spectacular sunset. Too weak to stand up for an extended period, she would ask every minute or so, "Is it time yet, Dad?" She wanted to take a picture of the special sunset. At exactly the right time, I would so indicate and Stephanie would get up and take the picture.

And her sister loved it, too. While Stephanie and her mother tended to stay inside, her sister and I explored the area and swam in the ocean, which she loved. But, after a time, she would always ask to return to the condo. She seemed to want to be near Stephanie. And she made a point of spending time with Stephanie, whose energy level was low, and who would usually be watching MTV. All too soon, we had to return for more treatments.

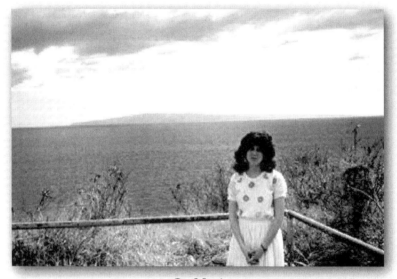

On Maui

The McDonald House in New York was tremendously supportive, particularly during this time. They constantly have famous people coming by, they have free tickets to shows, and they sponsor tours. Stephanie and her mother made the most of this whenever Stephanie could. She met Jimmy Conners of tennis fame, several Broadway stars, and on two occasions was on the opening of *Good Morning, America.*

I also did my best to support her efforts. With the help of his father, a personal friend, Peter Vidmar, the gymnast of US Olympic fame, sent Stephanie a beautiful note and a picture. I happened to be on the same plane as Red Skelton and asked him to do a sketch for Stephanie. I proudly brought it home, and Steph said, "Dad, I like it, but I can't quite remember who he is." I suddenly realized I was getting old.

March proved to be a tough month. Stephanie contracted an infection when her blood count was at the low point in one of its cycles. There was not enough time to get her to New York—infections spread rapidly when a blood count is low. So we took her to an upstate medical center in the middle of the night. She had to stay in the hospital one week to be sure the infection was under control. Word spread quickly among the doctors that she was there, and Stephanie Lemcke quickly became the "Lemcke case." A person with retinoblastoma and then osteogenic sarcoma is rare. During the week, a team of doctors dropped by only to examine her, since this is a teaching hospital. About the fourth evening, two more doctors came by, one after the other. I felt Stephanie had done enough for research and asked the doctor to leave. He did.

Back in New York, Stephanie wrote:

Dearest Marya,

Remember Nicky? I told you he was in the hospital and I called him mom, and he was twenty. Well, he died, I'm so upset. At least he's done suffering. Poor Nicky.

Did you talk to your employer yet? I hope you get the job. You'll be independent. Hey woman—can the fish borrow some $. Sure—here's twenty million. Buy a Corvette Sting Ray with green stripes.

And to her Spanish teacher:

Dearest Mrs. Wilson,

We got a new TV. It's HUGE—one of those 40" kinds. It has stereo speakers too. I got a dove. Did I tell you? I call him Derrick. I also got a 20 gallon fish tank to replace the 10 gallon. New fish too!

Marya likes this guy. His last name is Crum! So I bug her by say-ing "I'd rather be a fruitcake than a Crumb—and will you marry a crumb…Marya Crumb."

Well time to eat. I weigh 80, trying for 96. Write back,

Love,

Steph

And Marya, like a deep friend, ensured that Stephanie's picture was in the yearbook, even though Stephanie rarely attended school.

5/4/85

Dearest Marya,

Hi—I'm on the plane again. This time to Florida! We're staying at a classy resort on Amelia Island. I'll be back Wednesday. It was a sur-prise. I didn't know we were going until yesterday. My Dad had a big meeting there—and we're on our way. We're going to London in about ten weeks—groovy old chap!

I got my leg to bend 80 degrees—only 10 degrees to go. I weigh 84 pounds—good for me! Oh, I did quit my chemo. But it's not for sure the cancer will come back. They said there was a slim chance it would return.

Love,

Steph

In April, Stephanie had completed the second of what was to have been three chemotherapy cycles. By now, the side effects were becoming ex-tensive. Her veins were collapsing. At the end of that cycle, she declared that she was finished with chemo. She made her decision after a lengthy discussion with the doctors.

Later she wrote the following note about her experience:

Most of my friends tell me to keep a positive attitude—and it will be OK. It is not so easy. Anyone's opinion won't change how terribly worried I am. Prayers are better than opinions. Not what is being thought—but positive energy.

It's not what they think—Keep a positive attitude—things will be OK. To an extent, yes, but they have no idea what it's like. It's a whole other world. One where people suffer and die. You are not in New York to shop.

Thinking that her feeling would pass, we waited until the time for the next chemo and asked her again. The response was the same. We decided then to go to New York for another review with the doctors.

It was a terribly emotional meeting for all of us. We felt ourselves caught between different kinds of love. On one hand, we wanted her to experience no more agony from the effects of chemo. On the other, we were worried that stopping treatment would bring on a new malignancy. We had decided before that meeting that we would not push Stephanie, only let the doctors discuss it with her. The decision should be hers, unless she wanted us to make it for or with her.

After some discussion, Stephanie began to cry. I put my arm around her, told her that we loved her and only wanted what was best. The doctor said that she would like to see Stephanie take more, but could not say whether or not her treatments had been sufficient. Stephanie said she would not have more. We could tell she meant it.

For reasons still unclear to me, Stephanie then somehow met alone with one of the social workers who are assigned to work with teenagers and younger children at Sloan Kettering. I would not want to make a generalized conclusion, but some of these social workers were not helpful.

I tried as much as possible to keep them away from Stephanie. This was one of those coincidences when we did not realize what was transpiring. At any rate, for forty-five minutes, the social worker apparently pushed and cajoled Stephanie with those "Well, how do you feel about that?" intrusions. At the end of it all, Stephanie emerged furious and even more resolute. There would be no more chemotherapy.

At a later time, Stephanie would write the following about that incident:

This particular person had hair down to her butt and wore sandals every day—yes, folks, even in the winter. While still in the torture chamber of Ms. Hippy, I made the mistake of looking at my watch. How long had this been going on?

"I see you're looking at your watch, Stephanie."

So," I thought, "I see you sitting there. I'm proud of you for noticing and being able to verbalize by relaying my actions that are and remain to be none of your business."

"Are you going somewhere?"

"Yeah—out."

"What?"

"Nothing." Dumb jerk can't even take a hint.

Before Stephanie became ill, we had planned a trip to the UK to introduce the girls to those islands. With Stephanie off chemotherapy, the time was right to make the trip.

We hoped that by July, when I could get away, she would be strong enough. So we planned the trip. We made our way to Chicago and from there to Heathrow Airport in London. It was a long and hard trip, as the economy seats were fully occupied and Stephanie needed more room than was available for her leg. During the trip, an English gentleman gave his seat to Stephanie so she would have more room. As we exited the plane in London, he quietly approached me and said, "I shall say a prayer for your daughter." Tears filled my eyes.

We spent two-and-one-half weeks away. Stephanie loved it all, especially London:

7/31/85

Dear Marya,

Hi—we went to the place on the front (St. Pauls). It's huge and beautiful too. I'll show you the pictures. Dad got me an Olympus camera. The guys here can't be beat. Move to London! I said the same about Hawaii. So far we've seen Westminster, St. Pauls, London Tower (duh!) and Picadilly Circus, the part of the town where they're punky. We're leaving London tomorrow for Scotland, we see Ireland in a week.

Love,
Steph

We had visited Saint Paul's to find that Stephanie's camera was not advancing. So Stephanie and her mother went back and climbed to the Whispering Gallery, halfway up the dome. Later, when Stephanie became too tired, I carried her on my back around the Serpentine in Hyde Park. We didn't care who wondered why. We were seeing London.

Stephanie devoured it. In London, in a wheelchair, with each adventure she would say, "Dad, we've got to get a picture of that—closer."

After London, we visited Blenheim Palace, and the picture taking accelerated.

It was on this trip that Stephanie and her sister began to cement a fondness for each other we had anticipated. We were the common enemy in the front seat, they allies in the back. We were dumb parents, they concluded. They sang together, recited movie scripts, mooed at the cows, and bleated at the sheep. From England we went to Edinburgh, Scotland, where we shopped on Princess Street. I suggested Stephanie buy a certain dress, but she would not even consider it until she got her sister's opinion. From Scotland, Stephanie wrote Marya:

We got this postcard in York, but we are in Scotland now. They talk so funny here, haven't seen any cute guys—just got here. It's lovely here too. Fields and fields of cows and sheep and horses too. It looks like huge chocolate chips covered with green carpet! Castle ruins all over. We went to a ruined church.

Love
Steph

From Scotland, we went to Wales and then to Ireland. Stephanie said she wanted to meet the band U2 in Dublin. But clearly there was a second reason: Stephanie wanted to kiss the Blarney Stone, Ireland's eternal symbol of good fortune. From Wales, she wrote Marya again:

Dear Marya,

Scotland was truly interesting. The lake district of England has a lot of streams and stone walls, and of course, lakes. It's BEAUTIFUL! In Wales today we walked 2 miles around the city wall. Lots of cute guys in their Welsh wool sweaters!! We're going to Ireland tomorrow. Won't that be fun. In a boat. I didn't get to see my Welsh penpal. She had to work. I got to talk to her on the phone. I hope to see U2 and Bono in Ireland.

Love
Steph

And from Ireland:

8/9/85
Dear Marya,

I kissed the Blarney Stone today. We also went to see some crystal too. Oh yes, the guys—they're cute here too. Not as many around though. Didn't see Bono—better luck next century. Everything's green here— even paved road with lots of guys on the sidewalk.

Love, Steph

So we went to Blarney Castle, stopping at a beautiful old Georgian Inn near Mallow the night prior. We wanted to get to Blarney early, while Stephanie still had ample strength and the crowds were light. We arrived, and she headed for the castle like iron toward a magnet. The climb up to the stone, which is at the very top, is long and difficult. Her jaw set, Stephanie climbed up, almost without stopping, passing others on the way. When we arrived at the top, she promptly went to the stone, laid on her back, bent over backward and kissed the stone firmly. Stephanie wanted to live very much.

From Blarney, we proceeded to Cork, Waterford, Wexford, Johnston City, and the next day took the ferry back to Wales. With more ease, we made our way toward Heathrow Airport, staying in the beautiful village of Walton-on-Thames the night before our return. For the first time, Stephanie declined the offer to see some more of history, Hampton Court, which was nearby. She was simply too tired.

CHAPTER 9

A Short Respite

● ● ●

STEPHANIE HAD FREQUENT CHECKUPS AND blood tests both at home and in New York to keep a close check on the remission of her cancer. Her strength gradually returned. There were no signs of cancer.

After our UK trip, Stephanie and a friend did volunteer work at a local hospital, and she also worked for a friend in a local sewing supply shop. Since she couldn't move around very well, we also purchased a drum set, and I assembled the massive assortment of instruments in the basement. Our house had a large duct system, and those drums could be heard everywhere at the same decibel level. She had a picture of Bruce Springsteen, whose music she didn't care for, on the snare. If you came over to the house and she thought you were in a bad mood, she'd invite you down into our basement to whack your anxieties away on her drum set. It was louder than Derrick the dove, but we loved it.

In the late fall, after a long and chirping life, Julep, the parakeet, became ill and died. Stephanie proclaimed that Julep had entered into "birdy-heaven." We dutifully buried the bird and quickly acquired a somewhat less friendly winged creature called Petie.

Through deep friends, we were introduced to a "healing priest" named Father Swizdor. Wanting very much to strengthen her religious ties, Stephanie agreed to attend a service. Somewhat apprehensive and disbelieving in miracles, I agreed to go along.

Father Swizdor was a member of the Catholic Franciscan order. This order, based on the teaching of Saint Francis of Assisi, believes in peace and in harmony with nature. The priests are expected to take a vow of poverty for the service of others. Following several years as a parish priest in Pennsylvania, Father Swizdor became interested in healing. Just how he developed this capability is not clear to me. There is a story that his mother suffered a stroke at age seventy. He prayed over her as she clung to life. It was his belief that the family needed her with them for another ten years. She recovered and lived ten years, almost to the day.

Over time, his healing capabilities became well-known, and he spent about ten months per year performing healing services throughout the United States.

The church was crowded and we were relegated to a pew at least two-thirds of the way from the front. Shortly after the start of the service, a person near the front developed an uncontrolled coughing attack, which from the rear sounded like a side effect of emphysema. The priest momentarily ceased his address, left the pulpit, stood by the lady, and touched her. The coughing stopped. He returned to the pulpit and carried on where he had left off.

During his address, he gave examples of his healing successes. One such example I recall was a victim of a traffic accident. The person had been in a coma for some time and was near death. Father Swizdor told of visiting the person and praying for him. The next day, the person regained consciousness and, within a short time, was released from the hospital.

At the conclusion of his service, he invited all who desired healing to come forth, starting from the front of the church. This progression gave us ample opportunity to survey the scene. As things progressed, I became more and more confused. People would approach a long railing and await the blessing and, it seemed, the touch of Father Swizdor's hands. Behind these people were several suited assistants who would always position themselves immediately behind the person the Father was praying for as he worked his way back and forth. In about one of four times, the person would fall back, literally collapse, be caught by the suited assistant, and carefully placed on the floor. Moments later that person would rise, somewhat dazed, and return to his or her pew or leave.

The whole process was baffling to me. Being an engineer by training, collapse with the touch of finger or hand contact made no sense. My first reaction was that the whole thing was a set up. But as it went on and people dressed in garb from T-shirts to silk shirts collapsed with equal shock, I found myself forced to believe that something more than the first of law of physics was going on.

Our turn came, and I hesitated. Stephanie did not, and I felt compelled as a brave parent to follow her. So up we went. Father Swizdor put his three first fingers on the forehead of the man next to me and he collapsed like a folding chair. "My God," I thought. "What's going on here?"

My turn was next. The father placed his forefingers on my head, and I closed my eyes as he prayed. A sudden surge of something left that man's fingers and entered by head. I felt terribly disoriented and began to lose my sense of balance. I struggled for the rail as he was still praying for me, his fingers on my head. I opened my eyes to try to gain equilibrium and felt that I did not know where I was. As he concluded, I regained my composure and simultaneously felt that by fighting whatever he had for me, I had missed out on something very big.

The father went on to Stephanie. Full of emotion, I hoped she would collapse. I wanted her to be filled with whatever it was that this superhuman was giving out. All reason left my mind. I just wanted her to be well. She closed her eyes. His fingers went on her head. He prayed. I felt she was praying too. But she did not reach for the rails. She only closed and then opened her eyes, much more stable than I. When we returned to our pew, I asked, "What did you feel, Stephanie?" Her response: "Not a lot."

This was the only time I was able to attend a Father Swizdor service with Stephanie. It is as much a mystery to me today as it was that night. What I do believe is that some kind of healing was going on, even if temporary.

In the coming months, Stephanie would return several times to Father Swizdor both with her mother and our friends and sometimes with our friends alone. She never commented more on her feelings about faith healing or Father Swizdor. But knowing her, she was not one to waste her energy on something she felt was not worthwhile.

Our friend who introduced us to the healing services of Father Swizdor told me later that he prayed hard that Stephanie would be healed miraculously. When he later contracted cancer he said she was an inspiration to him. In fact, one of Stephanie's doctors who we'd recommended to him cured his cancer. But why, he would ask, was he so fortunate while Stephanie was not? He wrote, "If there is a benevolent God, how come she didn't get a cure? Did God put a young woman on earth, purposely, who was ill, to inspire? It's hard to say that God would create people, diseased, to help others. That's a tough one. But Stephanie was the kind of person who caught life, who didn't roll back into the doldrums, who swam, danced, and rode horses—to the very end."

In September 1985, having passed her grade ten exams, Stephanie entered grade eleven. With the respite, I attempted to catch up on my international travel. During a trip, Stephanie left the following note for me:

> Dad,
>
> Mr. Fonzo called and said he'll call back Montag (some German for you). Hugh Brown called and says he'll call you when you get back from Europa (espanol). And if your stupid friends don't quit calling—I'll unhook the phone.
> Love
> Fish

To return to a more normal life seemed almost unbelievable, and we relished it. Christmas was again special and important. We went through our usual Christmas tree ritual. But it was, we all agreed, a beautiful tree.

One of Stephanie's grade eleven classes was typing. We hesitated to have her enrolled in a formal typing class because, while she had learned to type somewhat, her eye-hand coordination was impaired when dealing with small print. She started, however, and to our good fortune, she had a Miss Becker as a teacher. Having been though some turmoil of her own, she understood all the struggles Stephanie was going through. Less than a year before she had met Stephanie, her brother had taken his own life. They developed an unusual relationship for a teacher and student. It seemed that in addition to Stephanie's respect for Miss Becker's teaching abilities, a second relationship developed, founded more in peer friendship. After Stephanie's death, Miss Becker said that Stephanie could have just as easily been one hundred years old rather than sixteen or seventeen.

During one of her health classes, the subject of cancer was addressed. A callous teacher asked Stephanie in front of the class what she thought about the subject. Stephanie responded that she had no comment and left the class crying, accompanied by Marya. Apparently, the teacher did not witness their departure. Stephanie discussed this incident at length with Miss Becker. She asked if she had done the right thing by leaving. Miss Becker responded, "You bet I do!"

Stephanie said, "Really?"

Stephanie also became a good typist. As always, with the right kind of support, she blossomed.

Following is her Christmas list from 1985, which we keep with other precious mementos:

CHRISTMAS LIST '85
(Good advice and convincing idioms)
For your (parental units) visual intake,
consideration, and deliberate, deep thought of
Fix the Walkman
Fix the High-hat
Decent Stereo (extensive equalizing, quadrophonic, dual cassette, etc.)
Bulldog
Preferably used additives for the existing drums
"5A" Drum Sticks
Preferably used guitar & amp
Water mattress (fish out of water are green around the gills)
$2,000 in cash or check made payable to yours truly

Lop eared rabbit
Completely cordless phone entirely for personal & private use
Fix the bathroom
Record vacuum or brush
Public Image—the album with Four Closed Walls
Electric kettle or tea service
Georgio cologne
Wind Song perfume
Albums: Yes
Tears for Fears "The Hurting"
The Smiths
Jon Anderson (of Yes)
China Crisis
That U2 video Dad owes me
a ½ way decent typewriter
Corey Hart's first album
The Cure
The Cult
Psychedelic Furs
Simple Minds
Blinds for both my bathroom windows
That pane of glass Dad owes me

We did not give her all she asked for, of course, but she made out well. She got her drum sticks, a cordless phone, a record brush, the perfumes and colognes, and just about every tape she asked for. And for balance, her sister made out well also.

With concern as to whether her bone cancer would come back and apprehension over the upcoming leg correction operation, we knew Stephanie needed positive lifts. I decided to try to get Ronald Reagan to give her a call to wish her a Happy Eighteenth Birthday. I used every trick in the book, including calling the White House directly, using what little political influence I had, and anything and everything else. It was all to no avail, however, partly I'm sure because the president gets hundreds of such requests every day. (There was a second reason, I found out. On January 17, the day before, President Reagan had entered a hospital in Washington for cancer surgery.) Nonetheless, the morning of her birthday, by overnight mail, came a beautiful letter wishing her Happy Birthday. It was signed by Ronald Reagan. She had a special birthday and that day wrote her friend Maya:

Dear Maya (hi chick!),

Thanks a lot for the groovy tape bag plus gum. The card couldn't be beat. So familiar was the word chocolate, but unexpected at first. I got a birthday letter from the President, Maya! Neat, huh? Marya says I only need one from Bono now! Doubt I'll ever accomplish that! I did finally get that promotional poster up. Proud of me? Other birthday gifts were real pearl earrings that have tiny diamonds in them, three albums (what?! What?! Tell me!!). Okay, calm down! In alphabetical order— O.M.D.'s "Crush", Prefab Sprouts "Two Wheels Good" and Simple Minds "Sparkle in the Rain". I love them all! You've probably heard of some of those.

We're all going out for dinner tonight. So I might get some more stuff yet. Too bad your birthday takes so long to arrive—haw haw— you've got to wait. Good things come to those who wait. Worse news yet. I've got to go back for surgery in February. My stupid leg got too loose so they're going to take the bottom part out and replace it. I feel like a god damn car!! Oh well life tends to suck at times!

Enough of this garbage. Please write soon.

Love,

Steph

And we did take Stephanie and three friends to a beautiful restaurant on her birthday. They sat alone in a section separate from us, but my concern for her well-being compelled me to check frequently. Each time, I would ask how they were and if they needed anything. I realized I had overdone my caring when, toward the end of dinner, all four came to our table and in unison asked how we were doing and was everything OK and did we need anything else, and were we sure we were OK. A few days after her birthday, Stephanie also wrote to her pen pal, Vicky Dimopoulou, in Athens, Greece:

> *Dear Vicky,*
>
> *Of course, I remember you!! Thank you for writing. My Christmas was decent. Hope your Season wasn't too shabby. I recently (three days ago) celebrated my 18th birthday. I got some real cool pearl earrings with diamond chips on the bottom. Also of course records! I like the "New Wave" so if I name them, you'd probably wonder about the mental status of the band members. For example—I like a band call Prefab Sprout but U2 is my fave. Do you like opera? My best friend's mom does—yuck!*
>
> *In February I am scheduled for surgery again. Hopefully it will turn out better than it was before. Cool huh? And since I can't ride my pony anymore we are teaching her to drive (it means pull a cart). Sounds cool so if you visit here, you can go for a cart ride. Write soon.*
>
> *Love*
> *Steph*

Stephanie did even better in school than she had done before her cancer. She was mature beyond her years and simply seemed to know what to concentrate on. Happiness for her was her Spanish class under Mrs. Wilson and typing with Miss Becker. Under the guidance of two excellent teachers, who became close friends, she flourished in these subjects.

I mentioned earlier taking Stephanie and her friend Marya to a Yes concert in Rochester. It was truly a spectacular show. We were relegated to seats too far back, but the whole aura of the show made up for it. This time, I stayed close to them, as the seating was temporary, the crowd emotional, and I wanted to take no chances with her deteriorating leg. As the show progressed, someone came around looking for whatever the paper is called that one wraps marijuana in to smoke the stuff. He had the same line for several people, "Would you have any— (whatever it is called)." Having no success, he worked his way down our row. Coming to me, he began the question, "Would you have..." —before even looking up. He then looked at me, stopped in the middle of the question, and said, "No, you wouldn't have any," and went on down the row. I felt amused, but old.

As the show went on, I saw a much different Stephanie than at the first Journey concert. She was truly enjoying the performance, but her actions were much more of an adult. She seemed less interested in partying around with the crowd than in listening for the message in the music.

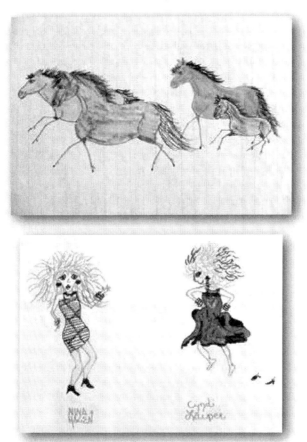

Maturing Stephanie expresses her joy through drawings

For several weeks, Stephanie had been complaining of headaches. We also noticed that her plastic eye seemed sunken in its socket. However, the headaches did not concern us, since every checkup, including body scans, showed no recurrence of any malignancy.

As she indicated in her letters, the condition of her leg began to deteriorate, possibly partly because of her riding. We knew beforehand the chance we were taking, and now it appeared that the doctor had been right. The strain of riding was too much for the adhesive holding the insert to the bone. There is no doubt in my mind that this was a price Stephanie was willing to pay. And we were too. Life is full of chances.

The operation that had been tentatively scheduled was now set for February 14. This was to be a comparatively simple operation, and we anticipated only a short break from school.

On the way to New York, Stephanie elected to write to Marya on an airsick bag and then on a napkin that she placed inside the bag:

Dear Marya,

Greetings from flight 432 on route to NYC. I'm in seat 15a and they're smoking in the row directly behind me—PU! I sort of distributed my entire weight on my headphones! And yes, they broke, never to be in one piece again. Dad's gunna get me a new one. Don't fall in love with any pervs, don't sit on your headphones.

Love Steph

And from New York on a napkin:

Dear Marya,

This is messy. I'm sorry but they dilated my poor eyeball and I can't see a thing. They're gunna CAT scan my brain. I don't know when though. I'll write you all about it if I don't have an IV by then.

Love
Steph

The operation was relatively short—four hours—and Stephanie recovered quickly. Although in pain, she refused medication. She wanted her head to be clear. The day following her operation, she wrote to her Spanish teacher.

> *Dear Mrs. Wilson,*
>
> *My surgery went well—or so says my surgeon. I hope your Valentine's Day was fun. They put me in the room with a VHS! But then they moved me to Room 510. My room mate is 13, y halbla Espanol solamente! Dad got us (me and Mom) some tulips. Pretty groovus? How's Jane? (Her doll, Rose Petal, reminded me—speaking of flowers.) So much for Spaghetti-o's for a while. I'm even having trouble keeping ice chips down—yuck! I should quit complaining now! Oh, one more—the food is as gross as ever! I brought my Spanish but I don't know if I can do it (estoy muy consado y borroso). I should quit Spanish huh? Dad also got me a new Walkman. It has a five band equalizer but the beat up one is even better. There is really not much going on here. They are threatening to give me some blood though.*
>
> *Sorry this is so short and depressing. It looks nice out. I'm here for two weeks so you can write if you want.*
>
> *Love,*
> *Steph*

Later, she wrote of the operation in her diary:

> *Ralph (Dr. Marcove) was so kind as to fix a few muscles so I could pick up my leg straight out. I heard them discussing what size leg to use to replace my crooked one. Yes—in the OR!*

Subsequent to her operation, the doctors gave Stephanie a brain scan to check on possible causes for her headaches. At first they saw nothing, but upon enhancement they detected an abnormality in the area of her eye prosthesis. A diagnosis would require a biopsy—yet another operation.

But since she was still recovering from leg surgery, we decided to bring her home. We did so eight days after the operation.

In discussion with Dr. Ellsworth the following week, we decided to have a biopsy done in Rochester rather than returning to New York. In my heart, I felt we were approaching the time to come closer to home. I felt that the cancer was gradually encircling us and that we were ultimately going to lose. I did not want her to die in New York City.

Only two weeks after her leg surgery, we took Stephanie to Strong Memorial Hospital in Rochester for yet another operation. She seemed to be placid, as if this was fate; my wife and I were very frustrated and concerned. It seemed we had entered nonstop surgery.

The operation was relatively simple. The doctors slit her eyelid and removed a sample of the malignancy. We knew the moment the doctor described the material that it had to be more cancer. "It was like cottage cheese, and there was a lot of it," he said.

Stephanie woke quickly after the operation and immediately wanted to know if it was a tumor.

We told her the truth—it was.

She did not cry, only became discouraged. The next day we brought her home while we waited for the diagnosis of what we were up against. As she was waiting to be checked out of the Rochester Hospital following surgery, she wrote a letter:

Dear Mrs. Wilson,

I hope everything is going well for you. Me, well…I am in Strong Memorial Hospital in Rochester at present. It's 9:30 a.m. I am waiting to be "thrown out". I'll bet you're wondering what it is this time (at least, it's my right eye anyway). Remember the numbness I told you about? Tumor action strikes again! Poor me! I am refusing any chemo. I guess its radiation again. They haven't actually said it's a tumor yet but what else could be growing in a socket muscle.

Mom says I should write a book—huh! She's even buying me a typewriter. Oh, I am sorry my last letter was so raunchy, I didn't feel too well.

I don't think I'll be back at "jail" (school) for a while. My leg is fine, they took out all 80 stitches while I was asleep in surgery yesterday. Fine with me. It feels great to be rid of them—they itched. Now I feel like running around the block! I'll give you a free copy of my book okay? And also tell you what I'm in for next when they tell me. We MUST have some Spaghetti-o's! Write or something, okay?

> *Love*
> *Steph*

We had begun to suggest Stephanie write a book. She had become an example for the nurses, doctors, and other patients in New York City and had become almost famous there. We broached the subject with some doctors on previous occasions, and they had urged us to have Stephanie write. Her stellar example, of course, was becoming too important to be lost. At first, Stephanie declined, but later she agreed and began a diary.

And while preparing to return yet again to New York she wrote of our animals.

> *Most roil kitty*
> *Beautiful black velvet coat*
> *Eating everything*
> *Black and white Gueff snores*
> *The Cutest little Gueff sleeps*
> *Gueff's eyes hardly close*

CHAPTER 10

Tough Decisions

● ● ●

As WE LOOK BACK ON our experiences, we have concluded that the worst is to not know. When you know, at least the problem is defined.

And so it was with the diagnosis at Strong Memorial Hospital. We were told after the biopsy that we would have the diagnosis in two to three days. I called on the second day, and the response was "tomorrow." The next day the response was the same. On the sixth day I called and was promised a response by 5:00 p.m. Receiving no call at five, I called to find that all the pathologists had left for the day. I felt like the slide from her biopsy had entered a huge sinkhole. Furious, I was able to contact a senior pathologist at home. I announced that I was finished with the people at Strong and that I would be in the hospital in one hour to pick up the slide.

A young medical attendant met me at the hospital with fear in his eyes. I took the slide, returned home, and took the first flight the next morning to New York.

Within fifteen minutes of meeting with Dr. Ellsworth at the Eye Institute, we had the diagnosis. Stephanie had a rare cancer called fibro-histiocytoma. This malignancy tends to develop as a result of extensive radiation sometime during the second decade following that radiation. It had been eighteen years since Stephanie's radiation at birth.

From New York, we hooked in a conference call that included Dr. Caparros-Sissons, my wife, and me. Dr. Sissons had received the diagnosis from Dr. Ellsworth. She sounded convinced that methotrexate, one of the less hostile chemotherapy treatments, would shrink the tumor. A complex cerebral operation would follow, because the shrunken tumor would have to be removed.

The reasons for Stephanie's headaches and sunken prosthesis now were clear. We were dealing with a growing tumor in her eye socket, close to her brain. We were confused, hurt, scared, and terribly frustrated. Stephanie had made it clear she did not want more chemo, and yet we were being told she would need this and an extensive operation in order to live. A crucial decision point had been reached. We agreed to bring Stephanie to New York in two days.

As I flew home, I felt as I had as a child growing up on a farm in Western Canada. We had always raised chickens, starting from incubator chicks. As they grew, they invariably escaped from the safety of the chicken coop. The plains of Canada abound with hawks, and inevitably a hawk would swoop down from the sky, pick a chick—screaming as much as its small voice box would allow—and casually flap its wings, reversing itself in the direction from which it had come. I would try to chase the hawk, throw stones at it, or attempt to hit it with a projectile from my homemade slingshot. I never saved one chick and would always return to the house crying, with a feeling of helplessness. This was exactly how I felt now. Some villain was taking our daughter. We were doing everything in our power to stop him, but we were merely throwing stones in the air.

The person we had come to rely on so much at home during Stephanie's second bout with cancer had moved. So now we had to try to replace her. We had no time to try before taking Stephanie to New York, so once more, our other daughter stayed with friends.

We met with Dr. Sissons in New York, and for the first time, I felt that we were not getting straight answers. Whereas with the sarcoma, chances of survival were stated in textbook fashion, now they were veiled in generalities.

I was sure Stephanie could sense the same. I drew Dr. Sissons aside, asking her directly if she would go on if this were her child. She was vague, but said that we had to understand there were only two options for Stephanie: go on or die.

We then met with Dr. Galicich, chief of neurosurgery, and Dr. Elliot Strong, chief of head and neck surgery. If we decided to go ahead, these doctors would operate as a team.

The operation would be very complex. They would literally cut out a box of a hole in Stephanie's forehead and perform the procedure from there. Spinal fluid would be drained, permitting her brain to recess toward the back of her skull, giving more room to operate. They expected that they would have to remove the bone around her eye socket. Stephanie asked if they could do the surgery without chemo. Dr. Strong said no. She asked if he could save her eyebrow. He said he would try but doubted that he could.

After some agonizing talks and tears, Stephanie decided to go ahead. Dr. Strong would be her lead physician. While she never stated so, I believe she decided to go ahead because Drs. Galicich and Strong exhibited so much compassion, competence, and perhaps most important, honesty.

The next morning Stephanie once more began chemo treatments as an outpatient. We stayed in a hotel in New Jersey near our former home. That night Stephanie was very ill, and early the next morning we admitted her to the hospital on an emergency basis. That evening, after her condition stabilized, she announced that she was going home. She knew she would die; she would not go on.

Did we have the right to force her to go on? Did we have the right to let her stop? What was our responsibility, and were we letting our love get in the way? And if we were, how? Were we being too willing to let her stop, or were we pushing her too hard to go on? Where was the truth? I felt I had no place to turn. If there was ever one time when I decided this book must be written, it was that terrible day in the spring of 1986 in New York City.

I turned to a good friend in Los Angeles. He and his wife had lost a daughter under similar circumstances a few years earlier. I called to tell him about Stephanie's current condition. I was reluctant to ask if he even wanted to comment—because in one sense I was asking him to be a part of our decision as to whether to let our child die. He courageously consented and asked that I call back in one hour to talk with both him and his wife.

I called back. At times, I became so emotionally choked I could barely speak. "What should we do?"

"Take her home," they said. "She is asking you to release her."

The next morning, Stephanie's resolve was equal to the night before. We prepared ourselves to tell Dr. Sissons of our decision when she arrived. (She usually came just before noon.) While we were out of the room for a cup of coffee, the doctor arrived—early. Stephanie gave her the decision. We found out later that the doctor—rightly or wrongly—put her under considerable pressure to go on.

When we returned to her room, Stephanie announced that she had changed her mind—she would go on. She was in the process of making a ceramic pot holder and positioning small pieces of ceramic in artistic shapes within the metal base. She would pick out long, thin pieces of ceramic and set them aside, saying, "That's a coffin; we won't need that one."

I have struggled with that whole episode since it occurred and do not know and never will, I suppose, what was right and what was wrong.

During this round of chemo, Stephanie wrote Marya:

I'm in Nuclear Medicine waiting for a galium scan. We have one and a half hours to wait 'cause of tech trouble. Then scanning takes two hours. I'm going to be home for a week starting Thursday or Friday.

They gave me methotrexate so I got really sick. It's 'cause I haven't had any for so long. I also need more surgery. I hope they get it all out. I'll look like Frankensteinette when they're done with me. Then on to plastic surgery or death (both sound as bad as the other) Dad got me a new walk-man. It's great. Cost $175 too. He might also get me a big $1000 stereo for Easter, if I'm good. I miss you. Write soon.

Love,
Steph

Easter arrived and with it a visit from our great former next-door New Jersey neighbors the Tighlmans.

Stephanie easily defused what could have been an emotionally uncomfortable experience. She casually discussed her condition, the possibility of her death, and the beauty of Easter. As the Tighlmans left, she hugged everyone and said good-bye. And that was what it would be.

Later, we received the following note from the Tighlmans: "The Easter baskets all melted on the way home—big puddles in the bottom of the baskets. Many thanks for your hospitality. I can't say enough for Steph's courage and control. Please let her know she has all our love and support, and as always we are available for all of you should you ever need anything. Our best to you all."

A few days later, after returning to New York for more chemotherapy, Stephanie wrote the following letter to Mrs. Wilson:

Thank you very much for the letter. The Spaghetti-o's guy was cute! I hope you don't mind the kitty card again. I feel all right presently, thank you. I hope all is well in there—your lives and the masses. Does Jane feel any older?

My surgery is in about three weeks. It's not going to be quite as drastic as they thought. THANK GOD! I'll have to get a special eye made.

I got the Walkman exchanged. The new one is fine. On April Fool's Day they played a U2 concert! They're no fools! Of course, with my new Walkman, I taped it on a hot tape. I got Mom to get me one from one of those dudes on the side of the street for only $1.00, bargain!

Our Easter was really groovy—but for leaving for New York at 3 p.m. Our old neighbors visited us—what a blast! We ended up watching my U2 video forty thousand times and I taped a bunch of stuff for Emily (the one I hang out with). I helped hide the eggs and Dad made me take a whole roll of film. The weather is great here, too, today was down a little though. I hope it stays like this.

Coloring the eggs was amusing.

You can come over and we can blast the stereo, watch videos, and eat Spaghetti-o's! I'll be home on the 11th. How was the pizza at Chuck & Cheese. Miss ya!

Love,
Steph

And to Marya:

Dearest Best Buddy in the whole world,

    Guess what? My face surgery may be OK. They're gunna see what they can do about letting me keep my eyebrow. I think I'm entitled to it personally. I've got the U2 video—sorry you can't see it for a while.

    Love,

    Steph

Two weeks later, she wrote her grandmother:

Dear Grandma,

    Thanks for writing! This is my new typewriter, pretty cool, huh? It does a lot, too. Nothing else has occurred lately. We had snow three days ago, stupid upstate weather. Today was 66, though. Mum hears on the radio that it was 10 degrees C in Dublin. So I know the guys in my favorite band (U2) are freezing their cute little hindends off! I also write to a pen pan Jill in Belfast, so I know she was in about the same shape.

    The chemo isn't too bad. I've had worse! I'd rather take this junk than die an early death—I feel there are a lot more concerts I really would love to experience, especially U2!! We might go to a real big show in New Jersey June 15! I hope so! I want to go backstage and meet them too and give them all a hug. Teenage thrill, I guess! If you visit and go to a concert…well, I don't know about that, now. Our neighbor brought some flowers for me, daffodils. They smell better than I can spell!

    This particular typewriter is groovy cause you can attach a computer to it. The computer has a dictionary in this case. Just what a horrible speller of today needs. As you can see, I don't have one yet. I can't think of anything else to tell you. My leg is marv, though. Write soon.

    Love,

    Steph

The expanding circle of friends who admired Stephanie included my business associates. With her new round of chemo, they smothered her with cards, letters, and gifts. Stephanie figured I had told them she was dying. I wrote her a letter:

Stephanie:

I cannot have you thinking I think you are going to die, because I don't. What it is, is pride and admiration. You see, people always look for heroes, particularly when times are tough. During the depression, it was Roosevelt and Will Rogers. During WWII it was Churchill, a singer called Gracie Fields, and MacArthur, plus some others.

These were all people who really showed their strength when times got tough. You see, most people appear about the same in easy times— it is the tough times when the really good ones suddenly show up and make the difference. Stephanie, you are one of those kinds of people. You have affected people you have never even met. Let me list some who call regularly in admiration. Rick Steber—Atlanta, John Strapach— Houston, Ed McKenna and Andy Woodbury—Los Angeles, Lee Topp— New Hampshire, Brian Rustom—Toronto, Luciano Carrera—Milan, Andre Cardin—Athens, Thomas Honse—San Paolo, Brazil, Arnoldo Semandeni,—Mexico City, Rene and Edna Grande—Manila, Bill McGaw—Singapore, Tom Freitag—Nanjing, China. I could fill another page. These people admire you for your courage, your positive outlook on life and the way you have beaten cancer twice—the fact that you have many ribbons, and yet have limited vision.

I don't brag about you—they ask and I answer. It is you who is the hero(ine). I am merely the proud father. I love you very much.

For some time I had felt an increasing need to do something special for Stephanie. Her mother was caring for her during her illness in a way I could never do. I felt terribly inadequate.

Stephanie had been a fan of the rock group U2 long before they had become famous. By this time, she had every tape they had made. During one of her trips for chemo a few weeks earlier, we had gone to the Sharper Image store. They had a magnificent stereo there, and when she expressed an interest, I simply bought it. We were not a wealthy family, but I had an empty feeling of not doing enough, and this was at least one way for her to enjoy some more of life.

I decided that somehow I would arrange for her to meet the band members of U2. I was not sure how, only that I would do it.

I made dozens of calls, but I was unable to make the right contact. Becoming more desperate, I contacted a friend in Cork, Ireland, and called another person in New York. Finally, on a Friday afternoon, six days before her radical surgery was scheduled, I got a call from U2 management in New York: We could have lunch with the complete band the next Tuesday in Dublin.

In a flurry of activity, we booked flights, arranged for the passport office in New York to stay open on Saturday, and did all else to pull it together. We left Saturday night and arrived in Dublin Sunday morning. In spite of having completed chemo only two days earlier, Stephanie made the trip in great shape, along with her friend Marya. We shopped in what seemed to be every record shop in Dublin, saw Malahide Castle, and even went to the Abbey Tavern in Howth, north of Dublin, for dinner.

On Monday morning, I received a call at our hotel from U2 with some of the logistics. We met with U2's administration personnel in Dublin on Tuesday—the purpose of which, I am sure, was to make sure that we were "real people." Having passed the test, we were driven south of Dublin into the Wicklow Mountains, where the group had rented an old home and were recording their album *The Joshua Tree*. As we entered, Bono spotted Stephanie and spontaneously broke into a song called "American Girl" by Tom Petty:

"Well, she was an American girl
raised on promises
she couldn't help thinking that
there was a little more in life somewhere else

after all it was a great big world
with lots of places to run to

Yes, and if she had to die trying
she had one hundred promises she was going to keep
Oh, yes, oh right..."

It only got better from there.

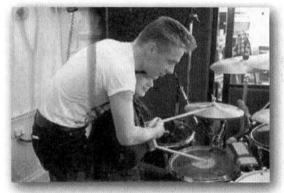

Drumming lessons from Larry Mullins

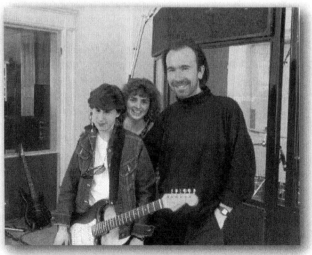

Marya and Stephanie – guitar lessons with The Edge

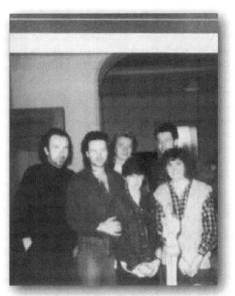

With U2 upon departure

We had lunch together, and Bono attempted to get Stephanie to sit with him on a couch. She was so overtaken that she declined, remaining at the table with the rest of the band. So he sat beside her there. After a time, Stephanie became more relaxed and was able to converse with her idols. Following lunch, the group led Stephanie and Marya into their studio where Stephanie received drum and keyboard lessons. Then Bono once again spontaneously composed and recorded a song for Stephanie, "With Our Eyes on the Distance, We Don't See What's under Our Feet."

"In the mountains deep and wide
In the song I sing in the sky
In the coldest night I'll wait for you

In the dance you danced for me
I will come and set you free
If you wait for my love
If you wait for my love…

Hold on for my love
Oh away, come away,
come see me, seven seas...
Oh fall in love again
Oh fall in love again...

A song for Stephanie
A song to set you free
In your eyes of clouded blue
Storm inside through to you
Heaven holds a place for you
I'll be there..."

Stephanie played the drums while Bono sang.

We continued together for several hours. Then a car pulled up unannounced and a person brought in a wood carving wrapped in paper. Bono presented it to Stephanie with his love. "God bless you," he said. It was a magnificent carving, made by an artist who also had his works in the Vatican.

Finally, the time came for us to leave.

Bono personally saw Stephanie to the car and once more said, "God bless you!" I thought that this would be the last time Stephanie would ever see the group. Stephanie had been quiet and reserved during our time with U2. When we returned to the hotel, I decided that the thing for me to do was to disappear and leave the girls alone for dinner. As they entered their room and closed the door, I heard them screaming and jumping. Thank God, and thank U2.

The next day we returned to New York. Stephanie and I stayed there, as she was to check into the hospital the following day for surgery. Marya went on home. As she left our hotel room, she hugged Stephanie and said, "I don't care if they take half of your face away, you'll always be my best friend."

The following morning we had the pictures developed and some enlarged and duplicated. I knew Stephanie would need continued diversion.

When we checked into the hospital, we found to our disappointment that Stephanie would be on a different floor with adults only, and that my wife would not be able to stay with her. From her diary:

Just because one is aged, does not necessarily relate them to being deaf. The staff likes to make very sure the patient—as well as everyone else who's not sleeping hears them. And if you are sleeping—well, you were. One chic was 87 and diabetic, among other things. They were arguing quite loudly one night around 10. She didn't speak English very well, but could communicate. I was hoping some understanding nurse would come to my rescue by offering me another room—a quiet one!

But there was this little miss helpless. The hospital procedure was not to her satisfaction. Breakfast came first—yes before you had a chance to wash. She was ringing the nurse at 7:30-shift time. She complained about the situation to me. I wondered why she didn't just shut up and eat first. So I asked her (politely). It seemed she had to take a shower first.

But Stephanie became an instant hit on that floor. She was a breath of fresh air to the staff that was used to caring for the elderly. Here was a person in trouble who had bounce and *joie de vivre*. We pasted on the wall the photos we had taken of her and U2, and soon we found nurses and assistants from all over the floor in the room. Word spread quickly and soon nurses from the children's hospital were up to see her. The pictures did what I had hoped they would do.

That night, a social worker came by to talk to her and go through the how-do-you-feel-about-that routine. After a few minutes, she came over to me and asked me to step outside. She explained that she was deeply concerned about Stephanie because she showed no fear of the extensive operation, no fear of death.

"Your daughter is far too calm," she said.

"Look, Stephanie is having enough trouble without helping you sort out your life. Please leave." She did.

The next morning Stephanie wrote her Spanish teacher:

Dear Mrs. Wilson,

I have radical face surgery in a few hours. I am quite calm, thanks. (Really I am, I'll tell you why later.) So how are you people and pets? I was home for a few days but it was quarterly week so I left you alone. Isn't this lovely paper! I only use it when I know I can write two pages worth, or when Mum brings it and it's all I have. I feel you are worth this awesome paper!

Stephanie went on to tell about her trip to Ireland, concluding:

My surgery is at noon. It's now 7:40 a.m. I am so thrilled that Bono wishes me the best. We got lots of pictures. Bono went wild with my camera. Hope things are peachy there. I'll be here for two weeks. I'm on the 9th floor. No room on the 5th. Please write. Miss ya. Love, Steph

She went into her surgery with her cross on her necklace and without pre-operative medication. She wanted her head to be clear.

After she was taken through the doors to the operating room, I leaned against the wall and cried for her. I did not know what would be left of our daughter when we got her back.

About midnight, after eleven hours of surgery, we were permitted to see her in the recovery room. She was barely conscious but knew we were there. As she recovered, she again refused most pain medication. She was beginning to go beyond the limits of pain and control it rather than having it control her.

Her recollections of that surgery are recorded in her diary:

They were stabbing me all over the place, and of course this is pain inducing. So I was indeed crying. They were needlessly telling me some usual crap like, "You're making it worse on yourself." How could it be worse? I could feel tears running down my face, and knew that would be the last time I'd ever feel them on the right side. Then everything went black. When I woke, I felt as if Jesus, or somebody up there had spared me my eyelids. I guess the muscles are still there is why. They'd stuffed packing from my eye socket to the back of my throat. Of course, while being sick, this did not help. I wanted this thing out of my way for it was causing me to gag.

So I stuck my fingers down my throat—to the nurses' dismay and complete disapproval—and proceeded to dislodge these clinging members. Having completed my mission, the nurses took it upon themselves to tape my hands down, telling me I couldn't do such things. "You can't do that to me, I'm 18!" Now that I think about it, why would that make a difference? I recall turning my head on the pillow, and feeling my skull crunch and grate together because of the change in pressure point.

Stephanie was convinced that she had been tossed from one bed to another in that operation. She wrote that before the operation: *I could pick up my leg straight out. That enthused me that is, until they threw me across the OR and managed to snap the muscle off.* Knowing the caliber of staff in that hospital, we concluded that this time her imagination had worked overtime.

We began to know and appreciate Dr. Elliot Strong. With time, we saw that his technical excellence and bedside manner were very much like Dr. Ellsworth's. Stephanie loved his no-nonsense honesty. After being with her a few days, he suggested she would be able to help others by writing a book and urged her to do so. A few months later, she would do just that and inspire me to do what I have done. She wrote in her diary:

Dr. Strong says I should write a book. He thinks I have a positive outlook and could help other people in similar situations. He said I've had a unique experience. All these people telling me this same thing—well I'm going to start believing it.

Shortly before returning home, she wrote Marya:

We took another picture of John sitting next to me. We also got another one of my medical assistant Jack (the wack), and another guy, Fred who's left the hospital cause he's gunna be a priest! He gave me a little bear before he left. I call him Pope Fred I. Cute bear! Since I'll be here till Friday, I took some time out to make you a duck. No, not exactly. It's a surprise! Blue and yellow and I won't tell you any more about it, curious? My idiot headaches have apparently let up! Guess a lot of people see pics of us and Bono and say "who's this? Your boyfriend? His apartment? And your friend?" Oh, you know I'd love that! But he's 26 and married. I'd just love to give him another hug. How I hope we get to see U2 again! Don't you just love Dublin, Erie and all in it? They messed up my leg— got to have more surgery on it after I recover. It'll be my seventh surgery. Miss you. Love, Steph

Two days after returning home from surgery, Stephanie wrote my brother and his wife:

Dear Aunt Lucie and Uncle Gordie,

    Thank you for writing. Yes, that U2 lunch was nirvana. This letter will have to sit around a while so I can get some copies of pictures made. I have so many people who want pics. I have pen pals in the UK. Dad probably told you everything so I won't say much. We got to play the keyboards on a song they named after our town! Nifty, huh? I also have the one and only copy. Who I mean by we is Marya, my best friend, and I. I couldn't eat—too shocked, I guess. Also, Bono was sitting next to me! I also got to be helped in some drumming. When we first got there, they were practicing, and dear Bono started singing American Girl! Nervy but practical—I was thrilled.

    The sculpture is in a special place all right—on one of my 33" speakers! Wonder what Bono would think of that. He also gave me a hug to beat all! Picked me off the floor! I want to move to Dublin. I want to get another hug—another 50,000! They're the most benevolent individuals to walk the face of the earth. We got a few things signed, too.

    My surgery did go as well as possible. So well in fact that plastic surgery isn't necessary.

Bono called the New York correspondent to wish me the best of surgery! That made me feel a lot better. Isn't he the most wonderful and caring individual in existence? Tomorrow we go to New York for a check-up. After this thing is all better, I get five weeks of chemo! Only five weeks!! Jesus does love me! The tumor was 100% dead! Marya said "It's not God's touch—it's Bono." Of course, I couldn't agree more but God brought Bono, right? I have to have another surgery on my leg because the muscle got torn in the operating room. I think they threw me across the room. It really feels gross because the metal is right next to my skin now. It burns when I bend it.

I'd better go to heaven for all this crap! In the song Bono says I will, I'll bring it with me when I visit, OK?

Write soon.

Love,

Steph

For the next several weeks, as she healed, Stephanie and her mother made many trips to New York. Before 1986 was over, they would make over thirty-five trips to New York City. In spite of it all, she was able to write and pass some exams at school. She wanted to go on to college very badly. On the last day of school, rather than call home for a ride, she walked, carrying her rather heavy electric portable typewriter.

Dealing with her added limitations (her operation caused her to lose most of her sense of smell), she proceeded to "do the possible." She and her friend Marya, after a training period, received their amateur radio operator's license. Starting in midsummer, they cohosted the "Rock Zone," a one-hour concert weekly on a radio station at a local college. Marya was designated "Miss Demeanor" and Stephanie "Womanfish." Stephanie ran the machinery, and Marya did most of the verbalizing. They concentrated on New Wave music, including, of course, U2. As the show gained attention, they received more and more telephone requests.

And she became an advisor. She wrote to Marya about a potential boyfriend:

Dearest Best Buddy Marya,
 Call Paul...or you'll be sorry or jealous or something. You've gotta have courage, pinkslip! Are you afraid of a phone call? No fears, no tears either if you call Paul.
 Love
 Steph the Womanfish

We spent a quiet summer as Stephanie healed. In August, we decided to return to Toronto for a few days. Stephanie wanted to see Lara, a friend from her early school years there. Stephanie wrote to Marya:

We left at ten this morning. Sat in the car for 4½ hours. This place is cool—it has a glassed in pool plus a TV, a bathroom, two beds...I sort of yelled U-U-U-U 2-2-2-2. Well maybe it's 2-0-0.
 I don't know if I'll see Lara tonight or what yet.
 Love ya,
 Steph
 P.S. There's a restaurant here called the Fish House.

She did see Lara the next day, and the meeting drew out a dramatic contrast. There was Lara, tall with beautiful hair, driving herself around Toronto. Stephanie was thin, her hair just growing back, with a patch over one eye covering a cavity that extended well into her skull, with little sight, little sense of smell, unable to walk well. Stephanie never said anything, but I somehow knew the meeting did not go well.

While her headaches never really abated, she went on to enroll in grade twelve. Together, we had determined a way for her to graduate and finish some senior classes during her freshman year at a community college.

She also resumed riding her horse—in spite of her leg problems. She had decided that as long as she was alive, she was going to live.

On October 7, 1986, another tumor in the same area was discovered. No chemo was recommended, only another operation. Stephanie agreed. She wanted to live a while longer.

CHAPTER 11

Beginning of Transformation

• • •

STEPHANIE AND HER MOTHER WERE visiting a friend who was in Sloan Kettering. He had been diagnosed with a mild type of cancer. They were in his room, discussing her own situation, when Stephanie grew depressed. However, after a few minutes of conversation, she said, "Well, Mum, enough is enough. I'm hungry. Let's go get something to eat." Once again, she did not bother with what she could not change. In October, Stephanie wrote a long letter to Maya:

Maya:

Did you know I've got yet another tumor? I have surgery on the 7th of November. Just in time to miss Peter Gabriel. I love him too! Now I understand why people think I should write a book…maybe. Are you for that? I wrote to U2 (well actually I typed a letter) and told them of my latest hell. This whole thing is really getting disgustingly monotonous not to forget annoying beyond belief. I'll be out of the hospital in two weeks. No chemo! No, it's not a relief, it's just one thing I don't have to go through, well deserved. But maybe nothing can stop this demise.

At the radio station, Marya and I have been promoted to "Wednesday night." Impressed?

Do you think I should write a book? Or do you think it's snobby, like I? I don't mean I'm snobby. I mean like I try to think. I am waiting to see what U2 thinks. If they think so, I'll see. I'd do anything for them!

In the name of love,
The Womanfish

A few days later she wrote Marya:

Glad you're feeling better! I am also glad you liked those tapes. Don't you just love my stereo's capabilities!

Better than that piece of trash I now keep in the bathroom to listen to while in the bath. I'm trying to get a CD player for Christmas. They don't seem to understand.

I think I had an anxiety attack the other night. I felt one half out of my body—spooky, scary. I thought I was going to perish. I got sick too. My face felt hot and my hands were clammy. Couldn't get a hold of myself. When I spoke it was like it wasn't my voice. I guess it was and is because they have been holding this upcoming surgery over my head. Now it's not even this week, like they have been telling me for a month. I went to see Spinny on Sunday. I dig her so very much! I didn't ride her, but did a week ago. My butt hurt for a few days. Out of practice. I sat around watching Red Rocks, and Unforgettable Fire video, to take my mind off the discomfort.

I have mellowed out, really, lately. Every time I get another tumor— I guess it works on my brain, and I get more tolerant. Zaps my energy supply, maybe—who knows? I don't get angry very much.

Mom got Rev. Hakes over here tonight to talk to me. Don't know why, but it couldn't hurt any. Glad you're feeling better!!
In the name of love,
The Womanfish

Of the anxiety attack, Stephanie wrote several pages in her diary:

I felt half gone. When I spoke, it was like it wasn't my voice. I thought I was going to die. I was nauseated, and it was hard to breathe, my heart was tolling as well. My face felt hot, and my hands were clammy—no abnormal temperature though. When the surgery is over, I wonder if I'll calm down any—it won't mean anything. What if another comes back? What to expect?

I do feel worried at times, though. I feel spaced out. It's like I'm half dead or something. All the doctors think it's nerves.

Her mother called the former minister at our church. He had experienced a tough childhood and therefore seemed to have a special understanding of what Stephanie was going through. They also shared the same sense of humor, which meant a lot to Stephanie. He quickly agreed to come and see Stephanie but was unable to come that night.

Stephanie later wrote:

Mom got Rev. Hakes to come over here. I said I guessed it would be an okay idea when I wasn't feeling well the other night. It couldn't hurt me any. I don't want to bother anybody with my problems. Poor Rev'll be sobered. I wonder if he'd like to hear some U2. He could watch the videos too, if he wants.

Reverend Hakes came, helped, but did not partake in U2. After that session, Stephanie wrote:

Well, the thing with the Rev. went okay. The forever present inquiry "How do you feel about that?" They always wait about what seems to be 5 minutes or so before they change topics and ask you how you feel about it.

I was describing my Saturday night experience to Rev. Hakes. I said I could hear things and not react. I could have if I needed to. He asked if it was just in my head, or my whole body. I said it was in my leg too. Now it's from my skull and my ribs. No fabricating either. I don't think it's (or was) one of those out of body experiences. I was afraid then and don't particularly appreciation this sensation.

It's supposed to be like a relief and peaceful to float around. I know one lady who was afraid she wasn't going to be able to get back into her body, so she quit.

And while she was still asking for advice on writing a book, she had, of course, already begun. She had taken the doctors' advice and responded to our suggestions. The first entry on October 25, 1986, went like this:

I rode Spinny today—for more than an hour, though it didn't seem like it. I was so happy to be able to do my favorite thing, which I hadn't done in about a year. Jenny said I made her sick because I haven't been on a horse since who knows when, and I still look as good as ever. There must be some flaws!

Our decision to attend church began to pay off. One week before surgery, she wrote the following in her diary:

I keep thinking about next Friday and surgery. Half of me says I'll be all right, my other half says I'm going to perish. If I average them, I'll be all right. It's times like these that you're quite appreciative that the church is praying for your person. All that good energy has to go up and do some good. If all those people weren't praying, I believe I would be a great deal worse off.

We received tremendous support from the church. While we were rarely able to attend, members constantly offered prayers for Stephanie and our whole family during services. Stephanie constantly received cards and letters from churchgoers. We even received special services for her through Catholic friends in Manila, Philippines. These prayers had a very positive effect on her. She developed a belief in heaven and a life hereafter, which played more and more into her approach to life as time went on.

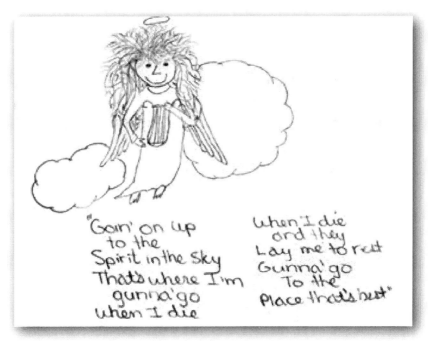

A sense of the inevitable

Her changing perspective became more and more obvious: An example from her diary:

> *I was talking to Miss Becker today, saying how none of my friends (the ones my age) understand how I'm not into drinking my brains out. Or at all, for that matter. Some of them do realize why I feel this way. I feel it easier to talk to adults sometimes. I guess college must be hell.*

A few days before her operation, I took her to the stables to see her horse. Her diary comments provide a perspective on the growing importance of that relationship:

> *Today I also went to see Spinny with Dad. I cleaned her up a bit and gave her four apples. She loves those, and french fries. And, as I*

recall, is quite curious as to what soda cans are, and what could be in them. She had tipped mine twice on a rather brutally hot day. I wish I could keep Spinny in the backyard!

I gave her a hug to signify the fact that we were going to have to leave at that point. As I did so, she rested her head on my arm which was then immobilized by the fact that it was squashed between her jaw and the stall. This same thing happened twice, because, after freeing my append-age, I had to hug her again.

I never really got tired of riding Spinnaker. I still love to.

A few days before her operation, she wrote:

I think dying is like a relief. Though I'm not waiting, or really looking forward to it. There would be so many people and things I know I'll miss. Like U2, riding Spinnaker, and going to Erie and seeing the hills and scenery. I love Erie, it's so beautiful.

As her operation drew closer, she wrote:

I was up because I was not feeling well around 4 and went to bed until 6 or 7 and couldn't sleep. When I was resting, I felt like I was being lifted up a little, then there was a tingling feeling like when you fall asleep and think HEY YOU—WAKE-UP! Weird, huh? I don't know what to think. I think I need a C.D. —this tape I am listening to makes me wanna cry—breaks my heart.

Before we left for New York, my mother called. At the end of her conversa-tion with Stephanie, she began to cry. After Stephanie hung up the phone, she said, "Hey, what's wrong with her?" She seemed to be developing an understanding and acceptance of the inevitability of her death—and, as a result, had problems with those who could not accept the inevitable in the same way.

CHAPTER 12

One Last Desperate Try

● ● ●

11/7/86

Today is the day I was supposed to have surgery. It will be this time next week I'll be in the recovery room. I can wait, believe me!

I wonder if it will be any different to be 19. Probably not since 16–18 has been such a depressing drag. I'm supposed to be in the COLLEGE OF MY CHOICE BY NOW. I wonder what will go wrong this year. No, I don't! Maybe I'll get lucky and get married! A U2 concert would make me happy

I got a 92 on my Spanish quarterly. Wow, I was so very shocked.

I must go and recurl my mop. It's getting too long. I would get it cut, otherwise, but they'll soon shave one half of it anyhow. I wish this wasn't happening again.

11/10/86

Mom called Dr. Strong because I was experiencing some numbness in my hands. He called back and thinks it's a nervous reaction. Any more of those and who knows where I'll be. What next?

11/11/86

THEY'VE SCHEDULED—well, they're trying to—a CAT scan locally. New York's too busy. They have one for Friday, but that's surgery day. They want another scan done because they've made me wait 5 weeks. Five weeks ago they said they could get it all.

I hope that's still the case, I hope they don't kill my one remaining vein. They've moved my scan up until 4 p.m. today. I have to do my hair today. Maybe we'll drive over and drape Spinnaker in her blankie, since it'll be 20 degrees soon. I was listening to Kate Bush this morning "And Dream of Sheep." It's so beautiful—and sad, kind of like that one "Holding Back the Years" by Simply Red. Don't cry now.

It'll be monumentally knarly to be doing the radio show again tomorrow night.

Doomsday. I found out from Mom while we were at the hospital that we are leaving tomorrow. I feel quite upset. We didn't get out until 6:30. And I was looking forward to doing the show. I'll have to leave a note for Marya.

I wish this wasn't happening. What if I die? I guess I'd go to heaven. I've never done anything wrong.

11/11/86

Dear Marya,

I didn't call cause it was late. We left at 9 this morning. Surgery is still Friday, but we have to go today to deliver the films from the CAT scan.

Miss Lott is taking care of my sister and the zoo.

On our radio show, could you please play some U2 and Kate Bush for me.

I'll be thinking of you, chick. I'll miss you too. Good luck with the show. Don't worry though, you won't need any. You'll do fine.

Write to me, okay. I'll write to you.

In the name of love,

Steph

11/13/86

The last 2 days have been spent in New York. Dr. Galicich said they might not have to shave my head. He came in today and relayed the information that he and Dr. Strong had been discussing the matter for

2 hours, and had reached a final discovery that they would go in from the top. Goodbye hair.

On the 6 hour drive to NYC, I wasn't feeling well. We had to stop and get a sick baggie out of the trunk. Unfortunately, I had to make use of the poor, defenseless baggie a few times. We stayed at Topps' apartment at 5th Avenue. Nice of them to let us use it, huh? I like to sit in the den and listen to their Pioneer rock system. Lucky I brought a blank tape! I taped 90 Sony minutes of WLIR 92.7. It's old, but it sounds nice.

The apartment is really big, and I want one like it. But now I'm in the hospital.

About 600 doctors have come in here demanding to see my defects. They might have to take a skin graft from my back, to use the muscle and blood vessels, to cover my brain. Only if they can't stretch the muscle across. It would be a 12–14 inch scar.

Radioactive seeds might be implanted, since it's not wise to administer any more outside radiation. I would rather perish than take any more chemo. This seed thing won't have any side effects. Hopefully, nothing of these sorts will be done. Dr. Strong said maybe not.

We went to a record store today, thanks to Jill, my Irish penpal. Now, how did she find out about this place?

Tons and tons of U2! There was so much stuff!!! I got a used one—another "Pride" record.

Going there made me feel better. I hope the next two weeks go fast.

The surgery may be 16 hours, if they need to do the skin graft from my back, then microsurgery. They're going to put me under the gas mask so it will be about 36 seconds of hell. It will seem longer, though. I'm going to be gassed because I have no veins left. The other time I asked, and the guy said I was too old. This guy is the chairman, so I'll get gassed!!

Dr. Strong was just in here again. He's out talking to my folks presently. He says I won't be out of here for two weeks. I tell him my radio show is suffering. He says he knows. I asked him if it would be easier this time. He says he hopes so. So do I. I hope God along with all else does too, for then—it will be!

STEPHANIE'S PERSPECTIVE FROM HER HOSPITAL bed was much the same as ours as we stood beside her. The operation had been delayed twice, and until we arrived in New York, we had not understood why. Once there, the picture that unfolded made it clear.

We had clearly entered the field of trial medicine—though no one had informed us. I suppose we should have asked more questions when no chemotherapy was proposed after the tumor returned so quickly. But I'm not sure what we would have done if we had known. The doctors were trying to save our daughter's life. It's just that the system seemed to have taken over without our knowledge.

There were not six hundred doctors, as Stephanie had written, but there were a lot, most with "Head of" on his or her name tag. The tumor had come back so quickly that Drs. Strong and Galicich had amassed a team of microsurgeons and others to stand by for any one of a number of alternative procedures, depending on what they found.

We discussed the alternatives with the various teams. First was the radioactive implant, which would emit low doses of radiation for a few months in an attempt to control the tumor. What would happen after the radioactive implant had lived its life was an open question.

There was a second, far more complicated option. Following this operation, we could take Stephanie to Massachusetts General Hospital in Boston for cyclotron radiation. She had received the maximum dosage of radiation in her first bout, eighteen years earlier. These cyclotron treatments, given by one of the most sophisticated radiation emitters in the world at that time, would expose her to highly concentrated doses.

But for her to receive these, the doctors would have to fill her eye cavity with flesh. They would remove the tissue, muscle, veins, and skin from her abdomen, tie the veins into her circulation system in her neck, and then run the veins and tissue up from her neck along the side of her head and into her eye socket. The options were terrible. Not knowing that we would be faced with such a complex situation, we were overwhelmed. And the doctors would decide on the spot which alternative to take based on their findings during the operation.

In the prior months, we had considered the question, "When is enough enough?" In the whole process, we felt pushed to go on, to try everything in the arsenal of medical technology. Her medical logbook had now grown to two volumes, about eight inches thick. On many occasions, we sensed that the technology of saving life had become so complex that life itself had become the victim of technology, not its master.

Stephanie was quite right when she wrote that, "Dr. Strong is talking to my folks presently." This is what he was telling us: "It appears from the CAT scans that the tumor may have penetrated through the tissue surrounding the brain into the brain itself."

I felt the options, if this were the case, were too much to ask Stephanie to handle. My voice and my whole body were shaking. "Please," I asked Dr. Strong, "If this is the case, perform no heroic measures." Calmly, smoothly, he agreed.

We then returned to Stephanie's room and managed to wear a smile when we said goodnight to her. Since Stephanie was no longer in the children's hospital, we, as parents, were not permitted to stay with her throughout the night. We tried our best to be allowed to stay, but the hospital policy was adamant: No.

We left her, and Stephanie wrote several pages in her diary:

I am the first case again because this operation will take so long. I am not going to take any preoperative medication. I hate them. They make me feel so queer and disoriented. I think they give them to you because they think you're too stupid to handle anything.

Dr. Strong says I should write a book. He thinks I have a positive outlook and could help other people in similar situations.

With all these people telling me the same thing, I am going to start believing it. Some, when I ask, laugh and say, "Do what you want." I guess they don't understand the situation.

It's about 8:45 pm. Mom and Dad just left. I wonder where I'll be—how I'll feel this time tomorrow. I so wish this wasn't happening. I feel like I'm going to have another emotional breakdown. But I don't want to bother anyone. Where's a U2 video (or more) when you need one. The pictures of us in Ireland will calm me down a tad. What would I do without U2?

I hope I feel better by Monday. Dr. Strong says I won't feel bad. From all the leg surgery, I felt bad then. Mom says I was okay last time. Why don't I remember? I do remember a little. I felt fine—but for a headache. I really must be worried, huh? I won't shut up about tomorrow, D-day.

(Later) I don't know what time it is. It's very dark, though. Now, maybe next time I write, it will be after surgery and not in pitch black.

12/9/86

It's been quite some time since I last wrote in this thing. Surgery took 17 ½ hours. I remember waking up and asking what time it was. 2:15 a.m. on Saturday. Last time I knew, it was 8 a.m. on Friday. I felt the pain in my stomach and knew they'd cut it up.

My parents came in to give me my cross. The nurse said they couldn't put it on my neck because of the tube in my jugular vein. "How about her wrist?" "There's one there too." So much for that endeavor.

When they brought me up from the recovery room about 9 or so, I was complaining about my stomach. It hurt to lay there.

In the recovery room, the chic was going to stab me with a needle. She did, of course. I asked what it was and what the side effects were. It was Vitamin K to clot my blood.

Time goes so slowly here. I kept asking what time it was and for water. They put A and E [ointment] on my lips. "What's that going to do?" I guess they were kind of chapped. They finally gave me a wet washcloth.

There was a lady there who said she remembered me from February. I remember her. It was leg surgery. She had said I was a model patient or something. How could she have remembered me? I had disagreed with her, anyway. I had been asking for water and when I could go upstairs every two minutes. Mom and Dad didn't remember her. They got a private nurse for me for three nights. I thought my guts would fly out of me if I continued to cough.

I didn't want any pain medication, however. They were telling me they gave me Demerol in the recovery room and I hadn't asked for any more. Even so, I recall I was in pain, but not enough to want any, out of fear. I am very afraid of drugs. Due to chemo, I am afraid of side effects. I'd rather put up with pain, than worry my brains out.

Some people do not understand this point of view. As one of the nurses was telling me something like, "Nobody gets medals around here…" for not taking pain meds. LISTEN. I don't want any medals. Good grief! What do you get with one of those? No love. (nothing.) That's not the point. There is a reason for my refusal.

I did, finally, take some Percocet to alleviate a rancid headache.

It so happens I suffered from spinal fluid leaks. I guess a couple of 18" needles in your back for as many hours will do it for you. They lasted for more than a week, I believe. They are gone now, though I suffered a migraine the other night. Pressure on your only remaining optic nerve is not my idea of comfort and relaxation, which I'm sure does not help the situation.

In the hospital, I had a few tubes implanted in my person. Yeah, man, two head drains, two IVs, one in my tummy too. It felt disgusting to have the one pulled from my head.

I don't recall the rest. The IV in the left hand came out. But the one in the right arm stayed for 11 days.

They also cut my ear down to my neck to get the stomach muscle in. I'm going to have fun waiting five months for the swelling to diminish.

Dr. Strong said, "If anyone on the floor has a level head, it's she." What do you make of that?

Ten days following her operation, Stephanie was back at home. We were able to spend Thanksgiving together.

And we made the best we could out of Christmas. There was no tree cutting, but Stephanie insisted on decorating the tree. As I took pictures, she became disturbed. "Why are you taking pictures, Dad? Because you know I won't be here next year?"

12/27/86

For X-mas I was so lucky to receive a CD player and four CD's. Now I am happy. But no, I received something more unique, yet ridiculous. A hernia! What next, man?

It so happens that the tummy tuck they did left my intestines no place to go but up. Up into my liver, diaphragm and my poor left lung. It is being smushed, causing me measurable discomfort.

This may afford me some surgery, of course, though I am hardly interested in such marked torture at this point.

I suffered another attack of the nerves on X-mas day. It wasn't as bad as the first one. Thank God! Still, it was not my opinion of amusing.

1/4/87

Now they want me to have another CAT scan of this hernia thing. It could be a tumor. I don't know if I could stand another. More surgery, I guess. If they radiated near the stomach, I couldn't eat any longer.

What am I going to do? It had better not be a tumor. I feel like an intensified lobe.

I'll bet the people in Rochester won't be able to find a vein either. I'm not in a foot vein rendering mood.

School resumes tomorrow. Mom asked me if I am going to go. I guess. I haven't been feeling much better lately. I always cry. I can't stop either, I have fear of going out of my mind and into Willard [Psychiatric Center]. Where it's so nice and quiet. Where there are a bunch of old ladies basket weaving.

Stephanie did go to school—and received, remarkably, honor-roll status for the first half of the year. It was the first time she had been on the honor roll. We were elated.

1/5/87

We were supposed to be in Boston today, at Massachusetts General. They want to clear up this diaphragm thing first though. Sure, prolong my suffering—make me worry.

Mom says I'll feel better after this is all over. I'm usually fine at night.

I hope this thing with my hernia (alleged) is no problem. It's starting to upset my stomach. I'm having difficulty sneezing as well. I can't get enough air into my squished lung. It hurts to yawn and laugh too. Mom says add sneezing to the list of things I can't do. The list is getting too specific for my taste. Too many things I appreciate and normal things are on it, i.e., I can't relax, my brain is in knots, and I wake up with a headache, so my worrying never stops, does it?

I also can't justify even one eighth of what's occurred in the last four years.

CHAPTER 13

A Time for Loving

• • •

THE ONLY WORDS TO DEFINE the situation seemed to be "out of control."

Time was essential if the treatments in Boston were to help. The operation in New York had theoretically removed the tumor. But from prior experience, it would probably return very quickly if treatment did not start soon after the operation. In our opinion, from the vague answers we received to our specific questions over the phone with Massachusetts General, the cyclotron radiation was clearly experimental. They said they had treated only sixty different cases. There was no established or even estimated survival rate. They could not define the treatment period, so there was, therefore, no established protocol. We were without a doubt in uncharted waters.

We were fortunate in that medical costs had not entered into the picture. As indicated earlier, in additional to regular major medical insurance, the company I was with had an excellent additional scheme for senior executives. Any medical costs beyond those covered by any insurance would be paid for under the executive insurance scheme. So, while the medical bills had been very high, we had paid no medical bills. We had, of course, spent a considerable amount of money for travel, accommodations, and help at home. But that was not, nor would it become, an issue. We were managing.

To begin such a long-shot treatment when we were now dealing with what had to be yet another tumor seemed illogical. Our feeling was that the cancer had metastasized even before her last operation. We had noticed the lump on her temple gradually enlarging, and then it retracted somewhat before growing again. In retrospect, we concluded that it was during this time that the cancer cells escaped to other parts of the body.

I could not see us going through more cycles of treatment in New York. Besides, it was the holiday season, and we had to think of keeping some semblance of family life. And Stephanie's birthday was approaching. And in all reality, if it had metastasized, the fight was over.

Through friends, we contacted an outstanding child internist in Rochester. Dr. Robert Emmans. I had a telephone conversation with him, explained our situation, and he agreed to help.

We took Stephanie for the CAT scan and ordered her files from New York for his review. Two days later, he called with the results. The cancer had metastasized. It appeared to be growing on her adrenal glands and possibly elsewhere. The mass was sizable.

Privately, over the phone, I had a long and terribly emotional conversation with Dr. Emmans. "What is right for a human body?" I asked. "When is enough too much…?"

"She has been through a terrible amount of treatment," he responded. "Maybe we can treat it, but it will be yet another major operation—and a difficult one."

"Am I fair in thinking we should not go on?" I asked.

"You are mature to fully weigh that option."

"Would you understand if we stopped?"

"Of course."

"Would you help us keep her as comfortable as possible?"

"Yes, you can count on me."

"Would you give her the grace to die in peace without life support systems?"

"Yes, I believe firmly in the dignity of life, and in the dignity of death."

The doctor asked if we wished to tell Stephanie ourselves, or if he should tell her with us. We felt it best that he tell her at his offices and carefully review the options with all of us so we could make the best decision.

Dr. Emmans told her the news directly (which was the only way she would have it), and he outlined the options. She asked several very pointed questions.

"Can you get it all with only an operation?"

"I believe so," he said, "but I cannot assure you it hasn't spread to other organs also."

"Even if you get it all, will it come back?"

"I can't say, but it may because this is the fourth time it has already."

"What will the operation involve?"

"It is a difficult procedure. We would have to go in from your back."

"How large is it?"

"About nine centimeters in diameter—large."

"If I don't have treatment, how long will I have to live?"

"That is a very difficult question," he said.

"Yes, but how long do you think?"

"I would estimate four to six months."

I could see that she liked this man; he was a straight-forward doctor. She wanted time to think. We agreed on a needle biopsy in the meantime, to see if radiation would help control the growth.

That drive home, like the one I'd made eighteen years earlier, remains perfectly vivid in my mind. Stephanie struggled with the decision. There were so many tears in my eyes I had trouble seeing the road.

She told us how terribly tired she was, how it seemed unbelievable that the cancer was back again, how part of her was ready to die, how another part wanted to go on. "Would Jesus understand if I felt ready to die?"

"Jesus loves you. If you want, he would be ready to take you home."

"Will Bono and U2 be disappointed if I stop the fight?"

"They would understand. Remember what Bono wrote for you in that song? Heaven holds a place for you."

Our emotions were all over the place, but by the time we arrived home, Stephanie was remarkably calm. She called Marya and told her she had cancer again and might not take treatments or have an operation. That night she wrote in her diary:

Now I know what's causing the problem. I am not sure I can relax. Even though it's a great relief not having to wonder, but to know it could kill me. Yes, again—the oblivious, notorious, abominable tumor strikes.

I need time to think. Part of me wants to die. I see that as a relief. I find it difficult to accept the thought that I would want to die.

Adrenaline tumors are rather durable. So if I did have surgery and radiation, it might grow back.

The other part of me wants to go on, endure the treatment. But then I think, why should I suffer more when Jesus would understand and maybe be glad to see me and think it was about time (too!)

It is causing me some discomfort at this point—being nine centimeter around probably induces this.

I'd really like to rap with God and Jesus. You're supposed to have this great knowledge when you're up there. I guess I'll find out about that soon enough.

Dr. Emmans said they couldn't remove it without major stomach surgery. This does not appeal to me at this particular moment in time. Ever heard that before? What do you suppose whoever said "moment in time" first meant. What is a moment going to be in?

Life isn't all tragedy. I'm going to a movie tomorrow night with Matt, Marya, and Dave. What to wear?

I'm not afraid of losing my mind any more. I'm expected to lose my life instead.

Months earlier, she had written: "I believe in reincarnation, life's not a dream. It means too much to be only one. I also believe that I shall go to heaven, and hope I am allowed to stay there."

The Dave whom Stephanie referred to in her diary was a friend of Marya's boyfriend, Matt, whom Stephanie referred to as "Wrestling Matt." Dave's mother had contracted cancer. Through this experience, I suppose, he became friendly with Stephanie, and, for a time, became a kind of boyfriend—her first and only.

After her needle biopsy, Stephanie wrote:

Marya and I went to the next town yesterday, so I gave my mind a bit of a rest. Keeping the knotted thing amused with using all my money for movies. Dad just came home with a very long-stemmed red rose. I said he could save it for the funeral. I wonder if anyone will attend. It'll probably be raining. Yuck—why can't I live to be old? How about 25? I thought I'd live after the eye radiation. So much for getting married. I don't have to worry about college—or graduating. It really didn't thrill me to any great extent to be honest.

I supposed I'd let them do the needle biopsy from the day we were told. I feel I'm at the end of my thread. No more surgery (certainly not that of the major stomach variety), no more chemo. We've got an appointment next Wednesday. The same day as our radio "Rock Zone". I hope I can take the news. It probably can't be radiated. It is soft though. I know because I got that needle biopsy at 9 a.m. today. Really vulgar experience. I refused their drugs. The nurse laughed when I informed her about my veinless state. So I underwent this procedure fully aware. I signed my own consent. But for some nerves in my back, I got some novocaine. I hate novocaine injections. Poor Lucille (the one who thinks my veinlessness is humorous). I think I squished her fingers off. I bent one of my mom's rings once. I don't believe I'm violent. I suppose only if I'm in extreme pain or hate.

Tomorrow night eight of us are going out to amuse ourselves. Reason enough for me to get my haircut. To hell with my lid collection.

My sister wants me to get a perm. No thanks, honey.

Stephanie seemed to be regaining her sense of humor and sense of balance in life. She wrote a great letter to her aunt and concluded this way: "Write to me—I'm not gone yet."

One of the most difficult things to do, or so we thought, would be to tell her friends. Once more, we were wrong. The love for her from her friends came like a torrent and continued to the end. Marya arranged for a page in the high school yearbook to be dedicated to her. Upon being informed, Stephanie remarked, "What if I'm here next fall and they say, 'Hey, Steph, you got a whole page!'?"

The big test of her relationship with her friends occurred two days before her nineteenth birthday. Marya arranged for a marshmallow roast at our house. We set up our TV and VCR in the living room and lit the fire. Friends began to arrive and, at first, the conversation was nonexistent, then slow. It gradually improved. My wife and I decided we should leave and went out for a late dinner. When we returned, spread out in our living room were fifteen super young adults, watching a movie, roasting marsh-mallows, and joking. Of that experience, she wrote in her diary:

> *It was pretty cool. We got "Porky's" and "Fast Times." We did eventually roast marshmallows. Dave took it upon himself to stick one of my choco-late chip cookies on a stick and thrust it into the flames. The nerve! Does no one appreciate homemade cookies? And if taking a bite of one and then saying, "Where's the dog?" wasn't enough. He said that wasn't how he meant it. I think he likes Gueff better than me.*

The day before her nineteenth birthday, she wrote:

> *I'M STARTING to get advice. When I tell them how my time is lim-ited. I get an answer—one in particular. This bit of info. Being that I should live each day as it comes. Don't tell me how to live, I don't need to be told what to do. It's no big deal, no huge catastrophe.*
>
> *I'd love to stay. But it seems I can't. Nothing can change that (but for somebody—Jesus). So why worry? Knowing me, this cannot be totally avoided.*
>
> *Since I shall have been around nineteen years as of tomorrow, we're having a 22 person dinner. That ought to be fun. And speaking of fun, today, I got a combo chicken/gorillagram! (too bad you can't include pho-tos in a journal). Alias a Marya/Kelly gram. Marya's forever talking*

about wanting to be a "chicken man." Kelly was also kind enough to send me some birthday balloons. It just so happened that I also received a dozen yellow roses.

That disgusting needle biopsy did wonders for my back. No longer ailing me. GREAT! I hope it remains in its relatively painless state.

Once more, her friends had come through. I remember the wonderful moment she was referring to in her diary. The doorbell rang. Stephanie answered, and in charged a chicken man and a gorilla. They showered her with hugs. The show went on for some time, and I took the opportunity to take many pictures. As they left, Stephanie took some photos herself. When we got them developed, we could see the tension in our faces. The tragedy was taking its toll on all of us.

The birthday party was as much as we could have hoped for. Her teachers, her friends, their parents, and Stephanie's boyfriend all came. The gifts were plentiful, many relating to fish. One friend gave her a hideous iridescent man's necktie shaped and painted like a fish. She put it on, her friends tying it. The table pounding began—"Stand up, fish. Stand up, fish"—until she could see there was only one way to stop it. She stood, gave a curtsy, which received a round of applause, and sat down.

After the party, Stephanie took a Tylenol because of her pain, and the group went to a movie.

A week earlier she had written in her diary:

Marya's gotten into inviting any senior woman she can possibly think of to the birthday party thing. First it was going to be four of us like last year. We're going to dine at that fancy restaurant. All 20 million of us. This ought to be amusing.

Once more, Marya had arranged a dinner birthday party for Stephanie. Many friends joined in at the restaurant for dinner and gifts. Once more, many fish-oriented presents arrived. This was not an inexpensive place, so I called the owner, a friend, and asked him to somehow gauge if they were ordering more than their pocketbooks could absorb—and if so, to send me a bill for the remainder. He did, and I concluded that from its size they emptied the dessert tray. It was a small price to pay.

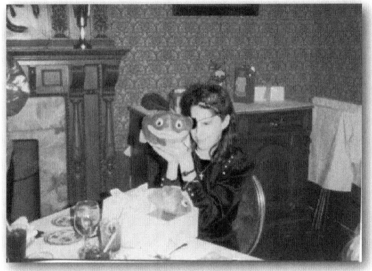

Fish Slippers for her 19ᵗʰ birtday

After the birthday parties, we reviewed the situation with Dr. Emmans. Radiation would control the tumor only for a time. The operation, should we elect, would be extensive. They would have to go in from the front. Stephanie said no.

It was a time for loving.

Stephanie wrote in her diary:

> *Before I found out what was wrong with me, I felt like I was in a box. I had never really felt that way before, or not that I can remember. Then when I knew what my problem was, I was still in a box, but it had a clear lid. I could see out but not get out. I have no idea why. Now there are only sides. Does this have some psychological benediction? I'm even actually hungry at times. I must be unbalanced upstairs. I cleaned my living quarters yesterday! You can see the floor!*

Wanting so badly to do more for Stephanie, I told her I would take her anywhere she wanted to go in the world. She declined, saying she just wanted to be home.

In February, I received an unexpected call from U2. They advised that they were conducting a major US tour beginning in late March and wished to see Stephanie in May in New York.

"May is too late," I said.

"Perhaps then we could meet at the University of New Mexico in Las Cruces, New Mexico, on April 10."

I was overwhelmed by their kindness. This group had now become the world's most popular rock bank. *The Joshua Tree*, which U2 was recording when Stephanie met them in Ireland, brought the group tens of millions of new fans. They remained as personally loyal to my daughter as she was to them.

Stephanie was circumspect but also very excited at the prospect of meeting U2 again, even though her problems were becoming greater, and she was taking prescription medication for pain control. But she wanted to go, so we made our plans. This time, she decided to bring her friend Maya.

But as we planned our trip, the tumor progressed and the pain worsened. Through Dr. Emmans, we made contact with a radiologist in Rochester. However, this man did not meet Stephanie's level of directness. Nonetheless, she began to take radiation to slow the growth of the tumor. On one visit, she asked the doctor point-blank how much time she had left. He responded vaguely, so she pushed for the answer. He finally said, "Stephanie, I don't know how to talk to you. You are too direct for me."

Stephanie wrote:

That doctor said I was too frank. He couldn't talk to me. What's he got against frank? Why am I hard to talk to? Mom said I took it wrong. I want straight answers—honesty—no secrets. Rob's [Dr. Emmans] like that—gnarly. This doctor, on the other side of the galaxy, is not. Makes me mad. Acts like he doesn't know.

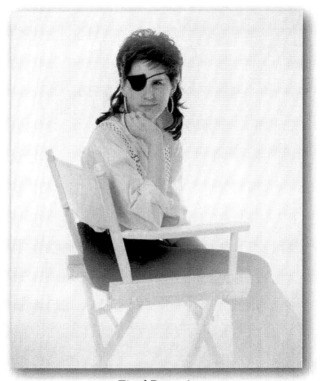

Final Portrait

For Valentine's Day, Dave had planned for him and Stephanie to visit friends near New York. She gave him a ghetto blaster, and he made a large Be My Valentine sign, which he placed on poles on the front yard. Then he gave her a heart necklace. And with that, they left for New York.

They had planned to stay two days, but by noon the next day, they were back. She had become ill.

Stephanie had set two conditions for herself. First, she would not accept any life-support systems, which she made clear to all doctors. Second, she would die at home.

In late March, the radiologist had an x-ray taken of Stephanie's chest due to her increased breathing problems. His reading of the x-ray: fluid was beginning to fill her lungs. He strongly suggested we admit her to the hospital. The next day was literally a blur of confusion. The medical staff attempted to take blood samples, but Stephanie literally had no available veins left. She wrote:

> *So they needed, yes, blood! I was being stabbed, wounded, and tortured by the world's worst, amateuristic, ego-inflated doctors in the entire complex. "You're making this hard on me, Stephanie." It's like, well, I told you, I have NO VEINS! My foot and arm feel like pin cushions. And this is QUITE PAINFUL! But show no mercy! Back again they were every half hour. I found this to be quite ridiculous and intolerable. I'd get so upset and act like I was hyperventilating—just calmed down and there they were again.*
>
> *They finally left me alone at about 11:45 p.m. I was so upset by all this, the pain medication wouldn't work.*

That same day, the doctor somehow concluded from the x-ray that the tumor might be wearing on a blood vessel. His concern was that it could break, causing her lungs to fill with blood. Even though he knew Stephanie wanted no life support, he asked if she wanted to be ventilated.

> *He suggested there might be a blood supply leakage causing the problem. If the blood vessel broke, it would inundate my person up to the throat, causing me to choke and croak. Therefore, would I mind if they stuck a tube down my throat in order to resuscitate me and preserve my "well" being. But "sticking tubes down my throat" didn't register to either Mom or I as ventilation. So I said it would be OK. Then he tells Rob [Dr. Emmans] that he thinks I'd take chemo too. I NEVER DISCUSSED THE SUBJECT.*

The nightmare ended the next morning. The other doctor had taken the weekend off, and Dr. Emmans, luckily for us, was filling in. He reviewed the x-rays and concluded that rather than being full of fluid, Stephanie's lung had collapsed due to pressure from the expanding tumor. He quickly released her from the hospital. And as he did, Stephanie again asked him how much time she had.

He asked her, "When will U2 be in New Jersey?"

"June."

"I don't think you will be here for the concert."

"Fine," she said. It was a straight answer. The wild ordeal was over.

As we left, I asked him how we could avoid getting involved with the other doctor again.

"As long as you don't ask for another doctor, I am by medical practice standard required to help."

"You are our doctor from now on," I said.

April 10 and the planned U2 trip was coming closer. My wife and I became concerned that Stephanie might not survive the trip. But we decided once more on the side of risk. I called the airlines and asked what facilities they had for continuous oxygen should a passenger need it. That raised flags very fast, and as they attempted to switch me to a passenger-service manager, I hung up. I was not going to have us blocked from going. I called a private service to find that a charter jet would cost $20,000. That route was out of the question. So we approached Dr. Emmans, got a letter that Stephanie was well enough to travel, and once more booked American Airlines to El Paso. With frequent flier passes, I upgraded us to first class.

We flew to Chicago and connected with Maya, who had flown in from Boston, where she was going to college. I had prepped the flight attendants about the reason for the trip, and they showered so much attention on Stephanie that she forgot about her pain and breathing problems.

The high desert of New Mexico was warm, and Stephanie was able to spend some time in the sun. She loved it and even got a hint of a tan.

The show was great, and at the end, I helped her backstage. She was almost too tired to walk, collapsing on the floor in the reception room. The room was filled with reporters who became quite confused. A few moments later, she and Maya were taken to a separate room for what turned out to be an extended visit with the complete group, as the press, including *Time* magazine, which would feature U2 on the cover the following week, cooled their heels. Stephanie and the group reminisced about our trip to Ireland, talked about their new album, the tour and more.

As it broke up, they signed a book for Stephanie. In that book are the words: "To Stephanie, the flower. Love, Bono, April 1987."

A few days after we came home, I asked Stephanie to watch a televised equestrian event with me. She declined. Shortly thereafter she asked that we take the riding ribbons down in her room. She seemed to be closing compartments of her life—reducing her world. It appeared that this was a part of her life she was finished with and could no longer enjoy. So she just shut the door on it. It hurt terribly, but we took them down as she asked.

Stephanie's diary became more direct, and her impatience seemed to increase. She became frustrated with those who could not deal directly with her dying. She wrote:

> *The discussions seem to end up the same. "Can I ask you a question?"*
> *"What?"*
> *"What do you think is going to happen to you?" Or "How do you feel about your...situation?"*
> *I guess "dying" is the plague word.*
> *I never asked them what they felt life without me is going to be. They seem to think I should have some idea of what it will be like and tell them. How should I know? I have no more idea than anyone else who has heard the tunnel and light stories.*
> *I called Maya last night and talked for 1-1/2 hours. She said she had no exciting stories and that I needed a vacation. FINALLY—someone agrees with me. Everybody else says give them a break. She says putting up with people is harder than the problem. It is.*

Finally, her pain became so great that she had to accept narcotics. It happened one night in early May. She had been taking more and more Percocet with progressively less relief. Finally about midnight, her pain became extreme. Her mother said, "Stephanie, you are going to have to go on something stronger." She finally agreed. Her mother called a local doctor and asked how she could get morphine. Totally against all regulations, over the phone, the doctor prescribed morphine injection at the hospital. It was a twenty-minute ride each way to the hospital and back, and when my wife arrived, the attendant became very concerned.

"Doing this is illegal," he said.

"My daughter is dying of cancer and is in extreme pain," my wife responded.

"OK."

In those forty-plus minutes Stephanie suffered terribly. I held her, trying to comfort her. She kept asking how long it would be until her mother got back. I gave estimates, being a bit conservative just in case she was held up for some reason. When she arrived earlier than expected, Stephanie dropped her shoulders in relief.

Stephanie began to be unfair to us, criticizing even as we were doing all we could to help. Then she began to refuse to do as asked and became very sarcastic. We were not sure what to do. I felt guilty about disciplining her since she had such little time left to live.

We called a social worker who had extensive experience taking care of the terminally ill. We described the problem. "You must discipline her," she said. "Everyone must have a code to live by and walls to stay within— even the terminally ill."

So we began to discipline Stephanie, telling her that in spite of her condition, she was not being fair. Within a short time period, she stopped being so bitter and sarcastic toward us.

Even though Stephanie was often not well enough to talk, her friends continued to come by in a steady stream. Miss Becker stopped by one night when Stephanie was in her room in bed and in pain. They spent some time together. Stephanie gave her a scenic picture with the following note:

Thank you for the HDYFAT hat [How Do You Feel About That, a hat Miss Becker had given her as a gift some time earlier] *and the gnarly earrings and for putting up with my raunchy typing. Furthermore, thank you for being one of my most sensible friends. Love, Steph.*

One of the positives Miss Becker told us she got out of her relationship with Stephanie was that their conversations never ended sad—sometimes with humor, sometimes with the sarcasm Stephanie loved so much, but never with sadness. On this visit, Stephanie was on oxygen and very weak. They talked about school, and Stephanie showed Miss Becker the yearbook she had just received and the full page that was dedicated to her. (Marya had taken the book around the school and it was filled with inscriptions.)

Stephanie was disturbed by some of the written comments put there by people who simply did not know what to say. One wrote: "See you next fall." Another wrote: "Good luck in the future."

"Why can't they be realistic?" Stephanie asked. A few minutes later she said, "By the way, would you like to sign my yearbook?"

As Miss Becker left, she said, "Well, I don't know when we'll see each other again, Steph, but if it isn't in this life, it will be in the next one." They both knew it was good-bye.

Stephanie started talking about her will. Piece by piece, she told her mother who she wanted to have what. Suzy was to get her typewriter. Karen was to have her fish. Marya would be given her earrings.

The time had come to select her grave. How do you pick a grave for your own child? It was, I believe, the most difficult act of all. In constant tears, I selected a shady area in a private part of an old cemetery. As I was looking, a bouncy squirrel scurried down a tree nearby and streamed across the ground, its tail high in the air. "There," I said to the superintendent, "right there."

A few days later, we noticed that our dog "the Gueff" was missing. A search throughout the area gave no clues. The next day, a neighbor came by with the news. She had found our dog in a nearby pond. She had apparently suffered a convulsion and drowned.

Stephanie took the narcotics in minor doses. And as she did, she began to ask for crushed ice in a dish. Before she got out of bed or as she went back, she would place pieces in her mouth and chew hard on them. It was not until a few days before her death that we realized what she was doing. To get above the pain, she was concentrating on breaking the ice with her teeth.

In the last weeks of her life, the list of friends shortened to those who could handle the stress of her directness most easily. We had purchased a special mattress for her to help ease the pain. It was unsuccessful, and it was lying on the floor in her bedroom when a friend came by. "Where did they get that?" questioned the friend. "From hell," Stephanie responded. Then she insisted that the friend try to prove her point.

One of Stephanie's closest friends told me later, "The last time I visited her, she was lying upstairs in her room, and she couldn't lift her head very much; but she could open her eyes and talk for a while. You could tell she was getting weaker, and she was saying that she just wanted to die then. 'When is it going to happen? I am supposed to be dying here—what's happening?'"

In the last few days of Stephanie's life, her mother became too exhausted to handle Stephanie's increasing needs. We arranged for two nurses to come in on a shift basis. When they first came to our house, they were terribly apprehensive, not knowing what to expect. After meeting her, they observed that they had never witnessed anybody with a more positive outlook than Stephanie.

One of the nurses was quite able to handle her direct approach. Such was not the case with the second. Stephanie asked her if she would live two more weeks. The nurse responded that she did not know. Stephanie's reply: "Well, you *must* have an opinion. I think you are older than my mother, and she has an opinion. Don't you?"

Stephanie was now confined to her bed, using oxygen continuously. We had solicited the help of a local doctor. On the morning of June 17, the doctor called at our house due to some complications Stephanie was experiencing. Stephanie asked how long she had to live. The doctor estimated ten days. Stephanie became very disturbed. She was ready for her next life and in too much pain for this one. Ten days seemed too long to wait.

As the day progressed, however, she seemed to feel much better. With help, and with her mother by her side, she took an extended shower and said over and over how good it felt. She took extra time to wash her hair. During the rest of the day, she seemed to have excess energy.

That evening, her mother and sister went out for some relief. I spent time with Stephanie, rubbing her back to help relieve her pain. "Will I go to heaven?" she asked.

"There is no way you will not be received."

She reminded me of the time, three years earlier, when she took a small record from a store without paying for it. (We later did.)

"That was a small detail," I said.

"I feel that I may have complained too much."

"Dr. Strong considered you a model patient."

"Can you get me my typewriter?"

I sat it on her bed while she started a letter to her New Jersey friend, Nga:

Dear Nga,

I am most sorry to report that I have little time left on the earth. Please bear with me a moment to explain. I am not exactly afraid to die, but it is strange to have to think of leaving something to which I cannot return. I'd love to visit you this summer, but for all we can tell, I have only two weeks left and I feel simply horrible. The only place I am going to go this summer is to heaven! No better place.

Enough of all that heavy material. I taped the Clannad I own. I hope it is to your liking. I would call you, but I am too weak. I can hardly breathe at times. I am on oxygen 24 hours a day.

She was unable to finish the letter. When her mother and sister returned, Stephanie was asleep.

She awoke later, and while her mother was sitting, holding her in her bed, she very quietly, very deliberately leaned back into her mother's arms and took her last breath. Stephanie died on her own terms, in her own time, in her own bed.

We congregated in her room, charged with love and emotion. I had never experienced another's death firsthand, so I cannot describe how I felt in comparative terms. But there was a feeling of tremendous energy, much like my experience with Father Swizdor two years earlier. Stephanie's body was still. But I could feel her presence, her spirit.

Stephanie's mother was holding her, and her sister was sitting at the foot of the bed. I kept pacing back and forth, first touching her "just one last time" I told myself, and then walking around the room in random fashion. I left the room, found the picture of her on her horse in New Jersey after winning her first ribbon, brought it into her bedroom, and attempted to show it to her mother and sister. I don't even know what my point was.

The oxygen was still on, hissing like a snake after its prey. I hoped against hope that my wife would turn it off. Finally, I reached over and turned the valve. It felt to me like the last step in her life, and, in a strange way, I felt like I was terminating that life. The hideous hissing ceased.

Later, I left the room and called the funeral home, asking them to come for her. As I reentered her room, I could still sense the tremendous feeling of power. I called back and asked them to come much later.

The next day, the first bouquet of flowers had the following message: "Stephanie is riding with the angels." It came from friends in Rochester who had put us in touch with Dr. Emmans.

CHAPTER 14

She Lives On

● ● ●

OVER MY LIFE, THE CONCEPT of life-after-death has come to my consciousness in three distinct steps.

The first step was disbelief. I studied engineering and learned quite clearly that just about everything can be mathematically formulated, particularly by an engineer. The phenomenon of the soul's energy surviving death had no place in my previous training. It was clear when the electrical impulses stopped telling the heart to beat, that bodily function ceased, and death came—all quite clear.

The second step, which was my first breakthrough into a new consciousness, came with my father's death and was confirmed by the death of friends and other relatives. It became clear then that life really does go on, in a continuous thread, with each of us touching the other. There is some of my father in me, so he is alive today. As I look at his and my mother's wedding picture in my study, I remember him, and he is alive again.

The third level came in the last phase of Stephanie's life and continues to expand to this day. There is a conscious presence, a feeling of someone being beside you, with you, and *within* you.

My first experience of this new consciousness came during one of my many trips by car to New York. I was on my way home after Stephanie's first cerebral operation. It was raining, late at night, and hard to see. I was crying as I drove, crying over the pain my daughter was in and the fact that I knew we were losing her. Visions of my childhood came to me. I clearly recalled standing near a tree where a robin's nest was built, a nest complete with family. A crow came by and, as the mother watched, picked up a young robin in it claws and casually flew off. The mother attacked again and again and screamed as I never knew a robin could scream. But the crow won.

And I felt like that robin. But then I felt a force, a presence, so strong that I kept looking at the passenger side of the car. It was my father. I had no vision of him, I did not see him, but I knew he was there. He counseled me, not in an audible voice, but with a message that somehow simply came into my mind. He told me that we were losing her, but that it would be all right. He created a sense of calm and then assured me of his love. Then it passed—and when it did, I became calm.

At Stephanie's funeral, the minister read messages by her two close friends and then accepted statements by those gathered. Her friend Karen wrote:

> *Those who were close to Stephanie know how special she was. Steph was warm and caring. Her concern for others will never be forgotten.*
>
> *Though she was obviously discouraged by her illness, she encouraged others through her sense of humor. I received many letters from Steph over the past few years when she was hospitalized in New York City. Each letter contained an amusing paragraph or sarcastic remark that only Steph could have written. Each letter brightened my day. When I got back and read these letters, I feel Steph near again, and I laugh with her. Our loss is heaven's gain. Now Stephanie can see well and run as much as she wants. She can breathe better and she'll never be in pain again.*

Marya wrote:

> *Dear Stephanie,*
>
> *You were my very best friend and I can't ever forget the good times we had. I had a trust in you and you always kept our secrets—we shared*

so many. You always were willing to do just about anything for me whether it was to go out with my boyfriend's friend or to lend me something.

Most of all, you were always willing to listen to my problems if others wouldn't. I'll never forget all the hours we spent talking on the phone or staying up late listening to the stereo or watching television.

You taught me a lot. Because of your illness, I learned that life is precious and should be cherished in great extent. I live every day of my life to the fullest. I only wish you could have enjoyed life, physically, the way I have. Remember the times I would tell you that I wished we could trade places? I really meant that. It would have made me a happier person, really. Before making a decision, I'd always take into consideration as to what you'd say or do. You were an inspiration and always of good humor, whether you felt well or not.

Well, Stephanie, I'm really going to miss you, you were such a terrific person, sarcasm and all. I'll always have you in my heart and all my memories of you will be cherished.

Shortly after the funeral, I received a letter from a very close friend:

If I were there, I would say some of these things to you in words. Since I am not, I will try to write them so they make some sense.

I was deeply moved at the funeral service yesterday. I was touched in a way that doesn't happen to me very often. For the first time, Stephanie's suffering and death made some sense to me. God was speaking through her to you and me and all those kids who talked about her. She knew what was important and learned it in a very short, painful life. I fear you and I haven't learned that yet. We chase after more money, power, and possessions, and because we are so tired from doing that, we miss out on much.

I was reminded yesterday how fragile is life and how important friends are and how hard they are to get and to keep. Russ, you were worried about using the church because you weren't a member. There were a thousand prayers said by lots of people for you guys during the past three long years.

God chose not to spare her life on earth but she and we surely used it to a great advantage.

It is so hard for strong guys like you and me to accept anything from others. But those people didn't come to that church because of your position, your wealth, or to impress you. They came because they truly cared about you and your family.

After the service yesterday, I tried to read the words printed in the church service bulletin. I couldn't finish, and all afternoon and evening, the song, "The Rose" that our friend sang kept running through my mind. My life will never be quite the same, and I have a feeling that song and her memory will come back time and again and I will act differently because of this little gal I didn't know very well.

There is only one other male in the world I would write this kind of letter to. I have two friends and it makes me proud to count you as one of them.

Peace.

Barry

A few days later, a letter arrived from a long-time family friend:

A beautiful June day—and with all your family and friends there with you I felt such a jumble of emotions.

While we did come in some small way to share your loss. It didn't work out that way. You gave us something.

I've never left a ceremony in such a positive frame of mind.

These past years must have been so difficult for you with the frustration of realizing that even after doing everything you possibly could, you knew it wasn't going to be enough. And in your quiet, dignified Lemcke way you lived with that.

Now you can visualize Stephanie completely unencumbered, I hope your hearts will be lighter.

Those bountiful tributes to her gave us just a brief glimpse of her strengths. So much to think about there.

So the day was one of thanksgiving for the life of Stephanie Lemcke.
It was quite a special day.
Love to you both, and your daughter

The day following her funeral, we attended the graduation ceremonies of Stephanie's class. The valedictorian spoke of Stephanie:

In the past week, our class has suffered a grievous loss with the passing of Stephanie Lemcke. Stephanie was a special person whose warmth, wit, and charm would often brighten our day. Everyone who knew Steph loved and admired her courage as she battled a mysterious and frightening disease. No—I am not sad that Stephanie has left, for she is going to a far better place, free of pain and fear. I am only sad that more of you did not have the privilege to meet Stephanie and to know her for the beautiful person she was and still is in our hearts. Steph's leaving us awakened me to the fact that life is too short and too suddenly ended to take it for granted. We will continue without Steph, and some day, inevitably, we'll join her. But we all lost a piece of our hearts with Stephanie.

At the end of her comments, she also announced that the graduating class was placing a tree in front of the school in memory of Stephanie.

The first diploma awarded was to Stephanie. With obvious pride, her sister stepped up to the podium and accepted the diploma on behalf of Stephanie.

After being notified of her death, many people wrote of their feelings about Stephanie. One of her pen pals wrote:

I do feel I know Stephanie personally. She had a personality that I believe could cross over any barrier, like communication by letter only—over the Atlantic.

If I can be half as brave as Stephanie in my life, I know I can face any adversity. I also hope that from having known her, I have captured some of her spirit. Her letters were always great to receive, always happy and chatty.

I know that this is a predictable thing to say, but Stephanie is still alive in all of us who know her. She gave us so much in life and is still giving it in our memories. I know that she is in heaven, charming the pants off of all she meets. I can picture her arguing with Mozart, forcing him to listen to U2, and promising to update his hairstyle.

Her typing teacher, Miss Becker, wrote:

I was trying to think the other day of how long Stephanie and I had been friends—our closeness made me think that it was years and years—but upon reflection, I realized that our friendship began not quite three years ago. As I put things mentally into place, I remember the beginning of the year—Stephanie (as her luck would have it) chose a seat at one of the few manual typewriters left and because the class was full, could not be moved to an electric one. Not only did this tiny person have to deal with a sight disadvantage, to say the least, but also she had to pound the heck out of the keys to get anything to print on the paper! But try she did and I knew from the beginning that her motor coordination was fine, and if I would get her to an electric machine, she would survive and learn to type. Probably by that time we were scheduled for the parent conference and the decision was made to have her work with me on an individual basis. How grateful I am and have been for those individual meetings. They were the ones where our friendship began and developed into one of the closest ones I've ever known.

I remember exactly the day that we knew we were really connecting— she came in, and I could tell she was somewhat down, she came in and start-ed her warm-up exercises, and I'd already learned not to press too hard for information. A few minutes later, before we started the new daily lesson, I ask if she was feeling okay—was anything wrong—she said no, not really, but why could people not understand her better? Evidently, something had happened in a previous class that made her feel isolated and alone—more so than usual. She sat on my left and I began by saying I didn't know why and I wasn't sure that I could understand either. I told Stephanie that the worst thing that had ever happened to me was my brother committing suicide the previous January—and that I knew it was really ironic that she was struggling all the time trying to deal with the desperation, frustration, and loneliness of a situation that was totally out of my control.

At that point, she turned to me to meet my eye, and I knew the connection was made. The irony still astounds me, but thus began our ability to communicate. In those daily meetings we talked just about as much as she typed, but as you know, she still learned the skill well.

So that was the beginning—we had many good talks and sometimes there weren't many words. Our senses of humor were somewhat similar and it was a great advantage in our talks—about a month ago when we were visiting—Steph was showing me her yearbook and talking about some of the things her friends wrote. It angered her that someone wrote, "See you next fall." I'm sure you heard her say it—I let her go for a minute, then with a little smirk I said, "They may not see you, but are you going to let them know you're there with some Twilight Zone sound effects?" That brought a quick chuckle and a smile and on we went.

On we went many, many times. Her friendship was very special to me and helped to give me the courage to deal with many difficult moments that were a result of my brother's death. We never spoke of Johnny's death after that first time, but the way Fani (my affectionate name for her) faced her life and the courage with which she did it gave me some of the strength I needed to deal with his death.

And now my dear friend Fani finally rests. I will dearly miss her, but my memories are rich and many.

A few weeks after the funeral, we received a call from one of the hospice nurses who helped us during the last period of Stephanie's life. She wanted us to know that as a result of her experience with Stephanie and the funeral, she and her husband had contacted their pastor and repeated their marriage vows.

Three months after her death, we received this letter:

I know that you do not know me, but my name is Tracy Guzzi, and I was Maya's roommate freshman year at Northeastern University. That's how I got to know your daughter Stephanie.

Although I never met her, I spoke to her on the phone a few times. I also knew a lot about her through Maya.

I am writing this letter for several reasons. One is to let you know that Stephanie was very much loved and still is. Her life made an impression on me that is hard to explain. I could write a million pages about how she affects me, but I still won't be able to find the right words to express myself.

Another reason I am writing is to express my and Debby Terenzio's and Sara Dixon's condolences to you.

The other reason I'm writing this letter is to tell you what happened at the U2 concert in Montreal at the Olympic Stadium. You are aware that we made a banner and gave it to a backstage roadie at the Hartford Concert. Although we never knew if the band received it, we do know that it made Steph really happy, because she couldn't go to the Meadowlands concert in New Jersey. Sara and I didn't get to see it either because scalp tickets were outrageous, about $100 for one.

We made another banner in Montreal so we could try to get on stage and make sure the band would get it. We had general admission tickets. It was so crowded and there was so much pushing, we ended up at the left side of the stage.

Every time Bono looked over we would jump up and down with the banner. The first time he came over to that side, he was singing—with his eyes closed! I was so mad that he wasn't interested in our banner. Debby kept saying, "Don't worry, he'll get it." I wasn't so positive.

He came over again and was looking at us. He pointed at us and motioned for us to give him the banner. I was so excited! Finally, after all of our travels, he would see the banner and there would be no doubt in our minds that he did. Debbie and Sara got lost in the crowd as people rushed forward to see him. I still had my hand on it and tried to give it to him. But I couldn't reach over the barricade to his hand. Bono asked the security guard to give it to him and he did.

At first Bono was very bewildered as to what this banner said, because we made it out of a full sheet. He was on stage fumbling with it to read it—well, now for the exciting part.

He read it and smiled—this big great smile—and hung the banner on the stage rail in front of 70,000 plus fans. The lights were on him and the banner. Needless to say, I went wild! The banner said, "Stephie Lemcke loves U2 and Amnesty." And the cameras were filming it. Maybe it'll be in their new video! But this is not the last of it! Bono motioned for the Edge to come over and he cupped his hands over the Edge's ear and said something. The Edge smiled too and started jamming on the guitar. Then Bono took the banner and wrapped it around himself and started spinning around in it! It was so long he had to spin 3 times until it was off the floor and around him. Then he went to the microphone, wrapped the banner around and finished the song—I think it was "Pride (In the Name of Love)" but I'm not sure because I was so excited I was screaming throughout the whole song! Then Bono took the banner, wrapped himself in it, and left the stage. He didn't come back for a good two minutes. He didn't say anything, but that's okay.

We went to the stage after the show and asked a roadie to get the banner back from the stage, and he looked for about 5 minutes. He said it wasn't there and that "the band already left." I wonder if Bono took it with him. Now we'll never know, but that's okay.

What that whole night meant to me and Sara and Debbie too, was that in a way we got to "meet" Stephanie—it was like she was there. But she was there! Bono didn't have to dance and to wrap himself with the banner. He didn't have to show it, standing above it, to 70,000 plus people for about three minutes. He usually just shows it to the audience, waves it around and that's it. I knew he did it for Stephie, for the same reasons we made the banner. Because Stephie was a special person. I never thought that I could be so close with someone whom I never met.

When Stephanie died, it didn't hit me until later. A friend of mine committed suicide about the same time. I felt sad about that, but sadder about Stephanie—my friend died a coward, but Stephanie died coura-geously, and I think happy. And I don't know if I ever could do that in those circumstances. That's why she'll always be loved and never forgotten.

Thank you for your time,

Tracy Guzzi and Sara Dixon and Debbie Terenzio

Stephanie had asked that we give Spinnaker to someone who would cher-ish her and take special care of her. Following Stephanie's death, I called her trainer and stable owner to ask his ideas. "I have exactly the right per-son," he said. The young girl he had in mind loved horses, but her family's income would not permit them to buy one for her. He made contact, and a few days later we received the following letter:

Dear Mr. and Mrs. Lemcke,

We are the parents of Jill Solfiell and would like to express our heartfelt thanks to you for the wonderful opportunity of allowing Jill to become the owner of Spinnaker.

Since Gary talked to us, Jill has been at the stable every day groom-ing and caring for Spinnaker. Over the holiday weekend, I also had the opportunity of spending a couple of hours at the stable and enjoyed mak-ing her grooming a family affair. Please be assured Spinnaker will have lots of "tender loving care."

Jill is nine years old and has been taking riding lessons for two and one half years. This past winter, she took her first blue ribbon jumping fences at Cornell. Like a lot of little girls, she always dreamed of having her own horse. To Jill, your bequest is a miracle and a dream come true.

Please accept our sincere sympathy at the loss of your daughter. Neither Jill nor we ever had the opportunity to meet Stephanie but she did ride one night this past year while Jill was in a lesson. Nothing could make your loss any less, but please know that you have put a spirit of faith and hope in one little girl.

God Bless you and your family.

Following receipt of that letter, I felt a strong need to see this little girl and to see Spinnaker one more time. So I called the mother and arranged to meet them at the stable the following Saturday.

When I arrived, the mother and daughter were there, and Jill was riding Spinnaker in the ring. Trying not to look at her, I went over to the mother and introduced myself. She said Jill had groomed Spinnaker extensively in preparation for the event. I suppose she was seeking my final approval.

Jill could have been Stephanie. Her mount was literally identical. She sat high in the saddle, her back straight, each movement done with care and attention. She held the reins a little high, as did Stephanie. And Spinnaker was responding as if Stephanie was in the saddle. Tears streamed down my face, but I did not want to leave, feeling that just maybe Stephanie was not gone after all. Later, I gave Jill some carrots for Spinnaker. Stephanie always brought Spinnaker either carrots or apples. Jill thanked me but said that she had already fed her horse several carrots. Why I put myself through that ordeal remains a mystery to me. Maybe I wanted to assure myself that I had done as Stephanie wished.

Three years after the death of Stephanie, while I was first writing this book, I invited a group of Stephanie's friends over to the house. I knew that, as a father, I could never fully see my daughter in the way others did. One thing was mentioned over and over again: Stephanie's boldness and how that boldness inspired those around her.

One of her childhood friends told a story:

"I remember walking down to the convenience store down around the corner. And Stephanie and I were on our way back—we had just got some Cokes, some candy, stuff like that—and she was telling me how she was a good runner. And I thought, 'Well, that's great, but I can run fast, too.' And she goes, 'Let's race.' That was a shock to me—a girl, challenging me to a race! I thought I was a pretty good runner. Well, we ran about a quarter of a mile to her house, and I got whipped—I mean, I was buried in the dust."

She was a person who could stand up to a challenge and who could create a challenge and overcome it.

I looked at how Stephanie approached things: if she wanted it, she'd go for it, she'd get it. Or if she couldn't get it, she'd do her damnedest, put in 150 percent—and that's a good hundred percent more than most people do. I pursued my career in large part because of Stephanie. I give her a lot of credit too for allowing me to do that, for not getting caught up with the fads, the stereotypes of our age. Stephanie allowed me to reflect on things in a deeper level than I could have if I didn't know her. I want to go after things to the degree that Stephanie did.

However long she was here, it didn't matter…two weeks, two years, or twenty-two years. Like every fairy in every fairy tale, she always seemed to be fluttering about, constantly using blunt terms, saying the world is real. She made you act real.

Her mother, her sister, and I have had unique experiences since her passing. We had purchased a large audio system for her bedroom on which she played many recordings from the wide range of bands she followed, but particularly U2. On different occasions after her death with nobody in the room, the radio would spontaneously come on with U2 playing a song, so many times "In the Name of Love," which was her favorite. Over the years, I have suddenly felt the need while driving along to switch radio stations, to find the same song being played. Our home was originally equipped with servant's bells that as far as we knew had long since been disconnected. Shortly after her death, those bells, which were at that point in the attic, began to ring. In all our prior years we had never heard those bells ring. The light in a bathroom flickered randomly. That went on for years, seemingly doing so at critical times, such as when the house was finally sold.

Stephanie's monument is both formal and informal, like she was. The front is quite formal with a proper border. On the back, a little like a trick, are reproductions of sketches she did of horses in every conceivable position: running, jumping, grazing, and rolling. Sprinkled among them, mostly on their tails, are several U2s. On the front, below the name Stephanie Anne Lemcke, are words from the U2 song "Bad": *If I Could I Would.*

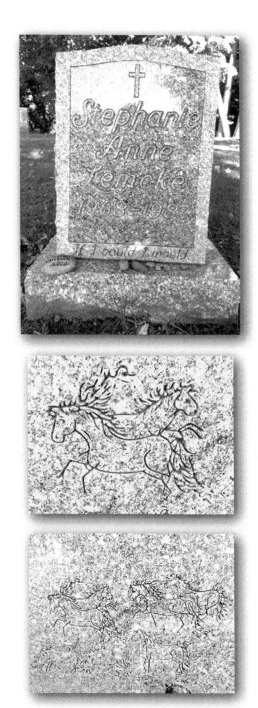

EPILOGUE
A DOZEN LESSONS

● ● ●

I WANT THIS BOOK TO help other cancer victims and families of victims throughout the ordeal. As I lived through this experience, I learned several lessons that, in my opinion, are important to share. Some of these lessons may apply to others, and some may not. Each one was important to me and all would have been more valuable if I had known them earlier.

Lesson 1: Seek the Truth—and Be Truthful

In almost all instances, we found Stephanie's doctors to be open and very honest. Sometimes, however, we found that we had to ask additional questions to get the complete story. I do not know why this is, but perhaps some doctors feel that if the patient or family wants to know more, they will ask. We did find people in similar situations who simply did not want to know the whole story. We even experienced one mother who did not want to speak to the doctors at all. We were best able to handle the situation when we had the complete picture of what we were facing. In Stephanie's case, she had a very strong desire to know and had no patience for those who were not completely up-front.

When I was a child the routine at a doctor's or dentist's office was for that person to say, "This won't hurt." And then it hurt like fury. Those days are long gone, thank God. In our case with Stephanie, we sought the truth for her and held nothing back. The result was that she knew she could count on us, and we all reached a new level of respect. Perhaps she was also different from others her age, but to her, truthfulness and open-ness were critical. For us, there could have been no other route.

Lesson 2: There Is Strength in Numbers—Most of the Time
One of the greatest benefits of the Ronald McDonald House and the brownstone, its predecessor, was the strength we got from other families. I believe Stephanie's mother found this particularly helpful when she was alone with Stephanie in New York. There is great value in talking through one's situation and sharing one's concerns and apprehensions with others. We did not go around seeking others to talk to. We sometimes found that those who did were not good company. But casual conversation more often than not resulted in a healthy and healing discussion.

Lesson 3: Love and Be with Your Kids
This lesson actually has nothing to do with cancer. But losing a child brings into very sharp focus the fragility of life and the importance of family. I know I too often sacrificed my family for my work. And it took the death of a daughter to teach me that simple lesson. My other daughter was clearly shortchanged in this whole process. In retrospect, we should have done more to help her through this difficult period of our lives.

Lesson 4: It's Not So Scary Once You're Inside
The jumble of emotions that comes with a diagnosis of cancer is terribly difficult to sort out. The initial reaction is that the victim is going to die, so we immediately face death rather than the disease that may cause it. It takes time to work through these emotions and face cancer as another ill-ness. But it *does* happen.

I found that the best course of action was to get the best information we could from doctors, friends, and other cancer victims and then *act on it*. Action in and of itself reduced the confusion and fear. And it keeps one busy and gives one the feeling that all power over one's destiny has not been lost.

Lesson 5: Don't Ask Questions—Make Statements
From time to time, particularly in getting into a cancer-treatment hospital, a lot of push becomes necessary. We met many families who basically waited for events to unfold for them. Time was lost, and their frustrations increased as a result. Each time we undertook a new treatment or went to a new hospital, I exerted extra effort to get Stephanie's needs taken care of. In doing so, it not only moved things along for her but decreased our own frustrations by the mere act of making something happen.

Lesson 6: Accept the Love of Others and Let Your Own Flow
Some are able to accept love and offers of help better than others. I suppose I was somewhere in the middle, although I certainly got much better at it as time passed.

It took some time for me to realize that people are not just trying to find something to say when they offer help. It is an outlet for them to satisfy their own feelings of helplessness in the face of a cherished friend's mortality. Accepting this love is tremendously uplifting. Take it in, let it flow.

Lesson 7: Draw Strength from Your Deep Friends
In the book, I referred to the difference between "friends" and "deep friends." Friends are those who offer help. I believe those offers are very sincere. However, the offers in their own minds have some prerequisites. They will help but within their own priorities. When one needs help, one needs it *now*, not when it is convenient to others.

Deep friends know this, and their offer of help is without preconditions. Draw on their friendship. First of all, when problems occur, they are usually of an urgent nature and cannot, or surely should not, be handled on someone else's time frame. Second, your deep friends expect to help.

Lesson 8: Don't Be Pushed Around
Many hospitals are teaching hospitals. When a patient has a serious or unusual illness, that patient is used to help teach interns. That is the way

it works. If one believes in helping people, then patients have some obligation to make themselves available to these interns. The amount of traffic any patient receives, I am convinced, is directly proportional to the uniqueness of the illness. In Stephanie's case, she became unique.

One must measure when enough is enough. Don't just accept that all the doctors coming through are necessary for the recovery of the patient. Ask why they are there. And when you feel you have done your fair share, simply tell them you have had enough. The word will get around very fast.

Lesson 9: Be Cautious about Social Workers

My experience in this area may not have been typical. Perhaps this was a unique situation in this case, but of the many she saw, it is my personal opinion that no social worker helped Stephanie. Rather, she helped them sort themselves out. If one encounters a social worker who is not being helpful, don't fool around. Tell him or her to leave and not to come back.

Lesson 10: Capture the Moment

When cancer strikes, hope for the best and plan for the worst. What that means is that each moment must be considered precious. If the victim feels good and wishes to do something, *do it—now*. Tomorrow may be too late, and that special time will have slipped by, never to be recovered.

Lesson 11: It Is Better to Know the Worst than Nothing

It should be clear from Stephanie's diaries that some of her most frustrating times were when she did not know what she was facing. I felt exactly the same. Waiting several days for Strong Memorial Hospital to provide a diagnosis was terribly frustrating to all of us. In a strange way, it was actually a relief when I flew the slides to New York and got an immediate diagnosis. At least we knew what we were up against. As in Lesson 5, getting to know sometimes requires unusual actions. And when you know, you will probably not like the enemy, but at least you know who it is.

Lesson 12: Go to Church

Even if you do not consider yourself a religious person, go to a place of worship. For me, it was a powerful help. I will not attempt a psychological analysis as to why—it just was. Through the church, we received offers of help. These offers alone made us feel better. Stephanie was obviously moved by prayers said for her, as were we. Through our church activities, she became a spiritual person, and religion helped her also. In fellowship, there is hope.

ADDITIONAL THOUGHTS

• • •

THE BOOK DOES NOT DWELL to any degree on my work life. However, I still struggle with whether or not I should have taken a leave of absence during the last phases of Stephanie's life. At that time, I was group vice president and on the board of directors of a publicly traded firm, and it was not clear to me how I could have just stepped aside for a period of time and left the position open. But maybe I should have found a way. As indicated in the book, guilt is the gift that keeps on giving.

In accordance with their desires, and out of respect for my former wife and love for my remaining daughter, their names and the location of our New York home have not been included.

ABOUT THE AUTHOR

• • •

Russ Lemcke established a Merger and Acquisition consulting firm in 1990 three years after Stephanie's passing. He is currently partially retired from the business. Russ and his second wife live on Cape Cod, MA.

Made in the USA
Middletown, DE
27 April 2017